The CEO-CIO Partnership:

Harnessing the Value of Information Technology in Healthcare

Edited by

Detlev H. Smaltz, PhD, FHIMSS, CHE, CKM

John P. Glaser, PhD, FCHIME, FHIMSS

Richard I. Skinner, MS, MHA, FCHIME

Terence T. Cunningham, III, MHA, FACHE

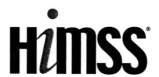

Supported in part by a generous grant
from Kodak's Health Group.

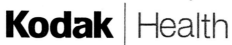

HIMSS Mission
To lead change in the healthcare information and management systems field through knowledge sharing, advocacy, collaboration, innovation, and community affiliations.

Printed in the U.S.A. 5 4 3 2 1

Requests for permission to reproduce any part of this work should be sent to

Permissions Editor
HIMSS
230 E. Ohio St., Suite 500
Chicago, IL 60611-3269
nvitucci@himss.org

The inclusion of an organization name, product, or service in this publication should not be construed as an endorsement of such organization, product, or service, nor is failure to include an organization name, product, or service to be construed as disapproval.

ISBN 0-9725371-9-8

For more information about HIMSS, please visit www.himss.org

Editors

Detlev H. (Herb) Smaltz, PhD, FHIMSS, CHE, CKM, has a dual appointment at the University of Alabama at Birmingham (UAB) Health System, a $1 billion-plus academic center, where he is an Associate Professor in the Health Informatics Program and also serves as the Chief Technology Officer. Prior to his appointment at UAB, Dr. Smaltz was the first-ever Chief Knowledge Officer for the U.S. Air Force Medical Service, a $6.2 billion globally distributed integrated delivery system. In previous positions, he served as the CIO for a 20-bed community hospital, a 301-bed academic medical center, a 5-state region, and a 7-country region. Dr. Smaltz is a Diplomate in the American College of Healthcare Executives and a Fellow in the Healthcare Information and Management Systems Society (HIMSS). He served on the HIMSS Board of Directors from 2002–2005 and as Vice Chair of the same board from 2004–2005. He earned an MBA from the Ohio State University and a PhD from Florida State University.

John P. Glaser, PhD, FCHIME, FHIMSS, is Vice-President and Chief Information Officer, Partners HealthCare System, Inc. Dr. Glaser was the founding chairman of the College of Healthcare Information Management Executives (CHIME) and is past chair of HIMSS. He is a fellow of HIMSS, CHIME and the American College of Medical Informatics. He has been awarded the John Gall Award for Healthcare CIO of the Year. CHIME has established a scholarship in Dr. Glaser's name. He was a recipient of *CIO Magazine's* 20/20 Vision Award. His organization, Partners HealthCare, has received several industry awards for its effective and innovative use of information technology. Dr. Glaser is on the editorial boards of *CIO Magazine, Healthcare Informatics, Journal of Biomedical Informatics,* and *Journal of Healthcare Information Management.* He has published over 80 articles and two books on the strategic application of information technology in healthcare. He holds a PhD in healthcare information systems from the University of Minnesota.

Richard I. Skinner, MS, MHA, FCHIME, is Vice President-IS and CIO for the Providence Health System, a $4 billion organization that operates 18 hospitals and a health plan with over 500,000 members, employs over 400 physicians, and manages numerous home health and long term care businesses across the four western states. Mr. Skinner has over 20 years' experience in healthcare information systems, including positions as the CIO for hospitals, a medical research laboratory, and project manager for the development and implementation of the Department of Defense's global medical information system. He was the recipient in 1994 of the Healthcare Information Executives Forum Crystal Award for Excellence. He received the John Gall Award for Healthcare CIO of the Year at the 2002 Annual HIMSS Conference & Exhibition.

Terence T. Cunningham, III, MHA, FACHE, is the Hospital Administrator for Ben Taub General Hospital in Houston, a 650-bed academic medical center serving as the flagship teaching hospital for the Baylor College of Medicine. Ben Taub has been listed as one of the Top 100 Hospitals in the United States. Mr. Cunningham has worked with developing and managing information management activities as a senior healthcare executive for over 30 years. His assignments included the U.S. Air Force Medical Service at various hospitals and headquarters and Johns Hopkins Hospital. He has written and lectured extensively on total quality management and using continuous process improvement and continuous cost improvement in hospitals. Mr. Cunningham graduated with a BS in microbiology from California State University, Long Beach and earned a masters in hospital administration from George Washington University in Washington, DC.

Contributors

Joseph E. Boyd, MBA, has over 20 years of information technology experience with Electronic Data Systems, KPMG Peat Marwick, GTE and Perot Systems. At Perot Systems, Mr. Boyd held a variety of positions from 1990 to 1994, when he was named Vice President and General Manager for the Healthcare Industry practice. In 1997, Mr. Boyd was promoted to Executive Vice President and General Manager for Perot Systems North American operations, directing over 4,000 employees in a $600 million business that included seven industry verticals. Mr. Boyd retired from Perot Systems in 2001 but continues to be involved in the industry, providing management consulting services through his own firm, Boyd Consulting. Mr. Boyd also serves as the Chairman of Healthlink Incorporated. He holds a BA in history and an MBA from Mississippi State University.

Russell P. Branzell, CHE, FHIMSS, is the Chief Information Officer and Vice President of Information Services for Poudre Valley Health System in Fort Collins, Colorado, a "Most Wired"/"Most Wireless" health system. Under Mr. Branzell's leadership, Poudre Valley also earned *Information Week* magazine's Top 500 Award for innovative technology usage and also received the Business Technology Optimization Excellence Award for IT Governance Best Practices.

Prior to joining Poudre Valley, Mr. Branzell served in numerous leadership positions at Sisters of Mercy Health System based in St. Louis, Missouri, where his positions included Regional Deputy CIO, Corporate Executive Director and various director-level assignments. He also held numerous CIO positions during his 13 years in the U.S. Air Force. He is a Fellow in HIMSS and a board certified Diplomate in the American College of Healthcare Executives.

Randy Carpenter, MSHI, CPHIMS, is Senior Vice President and Chief Information Officer for HealthSouth Corporation. He has over 25 years' experience in various information technology management capacities and is currently a member of both HIMSS and the College of Healthcare Information Management Executives (CHIME).

Drexel G. DeFord, MSHI, MPA, FHIMSS, is the Chief Technology Officer for the U.S. Air Force Medical Service, a $6.2 billion globally distributed healthcare system with over 39,000 employees and 74 hospitals and clinics. During his 19-year military career, he has served as a Regional Chief Information Officer, a Medical Center Chief Information Officer, and has completed two tours in Southwest Asia, including Operations Desert Shield and Desert Storm. He is a Fellow in HIMSS, where he serves as the Chair of the Microsoft Healthcare Users' Group Board of Directors, and as an Advisory Member to the HIMSS Board of Directors. He holds masters degrees in both public administration and health informatics.

David E. Garets, FHIMSS, is President and CEO of HIMSS Analytics. With 27 years of experience in information technology, Mr. Garets joined HIMSS Analytics in 2004 from Healthlink Incorporated where he was Executive Vice President. Prior to that, he was Group Vice President, Healthcare Industry Research and Advisory Services, at Gartner, Inc. Before joining Gartner in 1998, he was with First Consulting Group where he was Senior Manager in Emerging Practices and also served as CIO of Magic Valley Regional Medical Center in Twin Falls, Idaho, for five years. He was a course director and served on the faculties of the College of Healthcare Information Management Executives (CHIME) Information Management Executive Courses for 11 years. Mr. Garets serves on the editorial advisory boards of seven health care information technology journals and magazines and is a HIMSS Fellow. He was chair of the HIMSS Board of Directors for 2003–2004.

David Hoidal, MHA, is CEO of UAB Health System, where he previously served as Chief Operating Officer, overseeing the daily operations of the University Hospital, the Callahan Eye Foundation Hospital and The Kirklin Clinic. Prior to UAB, Mr. Hoidal was the Senior Vice President and Chief Operating Officer of Tulane University Hospital and Clinics in Louisiana. Prior to joining Tulane, he served as CEO of DePaul/Tulane Behavioral Health Center in New Orleans as well as CEO for HCA Peninsula Hospital in Hampton, Virginia. Mr. Hoidal has received the HCA award for Outstanding Operations, has acted as an HCA Quality Assurance Surveyor, and has been named one of *Healthweek's* Top 25 Turnaround CEOs. He received his BA in psychology from the University of Nebraska and a masters degree in health administration from the University of Missouri-Columbia.

Walter R. Menning, FHMISS, is the Vice Chair of Information Services at the Mayo Clinic in Rochester, Minnesota. Mr. Menning is a Fellow in HIMSS, where he served as a member of the Board of Directors from 1998–2002 and Chair from 2000–2001. He is the 1997 recipient of the John E. Gall Jr. CIO Award for outstanding contributions to the field of healthcare information technology management.

Michael W. Murphy, CPA, has been President and CEO of Sharp HealthCare since June 1996. Sharp is the largest health system and the largest private-sector employer in San Diego, with four acute care hospitals, four specialty hospitals, three medical groups, and a health plan. Mr. Murphy currently serves on a number of healthcare boards and committees throughout the country and, locally, is vice-chairman of the board of directors of the San Diego Regional Chamber of Commerce and the California Association of Hospitals and Health Systems Board of Trustees. He also actively supports a number of San Diego organizations such as the American Heart Association, MS Society, American Cancer Society, and the Union of Pan Asian Communities.

Dennis R. (Denny) Porter, MBA, MIS, is a senior executive in Integic's Health-Care Practice Area. Throughout a healthcare career spanning more than 25 years he has served in a variety of business executive leadership roles, including Chief Information Officer. He is one of nine national leaders serving on the HIMSS Electronic Health Record Steering Committee. Mr. Porter earned a masters degree in business administration management information systems from Oklahoma City University.

Stephanie L. Reel, MBA, is the Chief Information Officer and Vice Provost for Information Technology for the Johns Hopkins University, and Vice President for Information Services for Johns Hopkins Medicine. Ms. Reel earned a BS in information systems management from the University of Maryland and an MBA from Loyola College of Baltimore. The College of Healthcare Information Systems Executives named her CIO of the Year in 2000. Her innovations have been recognized by *Computerworld* and the Smithsonian Institute with an award that remains on display in the Smithsonian's Museum of American History. Ms. Reel is a member of the Board of Directors for the Microsoft Healthcare Users Group, the Healthcare Information Systems Executive Association, the GE Medical Systems Global Advisory Board, the College of Healthcare Information Systems Executives, HIMSS, the HealthCare Advisory Council, and the National Alliance for Health Information Technology. She also serves on the State of Maryland's Medical Privacy and Confidentiality Advisory Board.

William A. Spooner has been CIO for the past 8 of his 25 years at Sharp HealthCare in San Diego. He has led an aggressive IT effort that has placed Sharp on the *Hospitals and Health Networks* 100 Most Wired list for all six years since the list was established. Sharp has been an early leader in EDI development among its payers and providers. Sharp was also recognized as an early adopter for its leading edge consumer Web site. Mr. Spooner is a member of the Healthcare Information Systems Executive Association (HISEA), the College of Healthcare Information Management Executives (CHIME) and HIMSS. He is currently serving on the CHIME Board of Trustees. He has presented the Sharp model at several industry conferences.

Rulon F. Stacey, PhD, is CEO of Poudre Valley Health System, a five-hospital system based in Fort Collins, CO. In 1999 Dr. Stacey received the Robert S. Hudgens Award from the American College of Healthcare Executives as the "Young Healthcare Executive of the Year." In 1992, Dr. Stacey was named one of 12 executives under age 40 "who have taken considerable strides to improve the cost, access and overall quality of healthcare delivery in the United States" by *Modern Healthcare* magazine. Dr. Stacey holds a bachelor of science in economics, a masters degree in health administration from Brigham Young University, and a doctor of philosophy in health policy from the University of Colorado.

Michael R. Waldrum, MD, MS, has been the Chief Operating Officer of UAB Health System since December 2004. Prior to that he was the CIO of UAB Health System since June 1999 and provided leadership and oversight of all Health System Information Services (HSIS) activities and coordinated IT and IM strategies for the entities of the health system. Prior to becoming the CIO, he was the Medical Director for HSIS, where he was responsible for directing strategic projects such as Physician Order Entry and Clinical Document Access (CDA). In addition, Dr. Waldrum also continues to practice medicine within the UAB Health System and is the Medical Director for the UAB Hospital Medical Intensive Care Unit. Dr. Waldrum received his medical degree from the University of Alabama School of Medicine. He completed his residency in Internal Medicine at the Mayo Clinic and then returned to UAB to train in pulmonary and critical care medicine. He also has an MS in epidemiology from the Harvard School of Public Health.

Contents

Preface

Ideas emerge serendipitously. At the American College of Healthcare Executives (ACHE) 2003 Congress on Healthcare Management in Chicago, my colleagues John Glaser and Rick Skinner were presenting on two topics near and dear to my heart: "How to Calculate Return on Investment (ROI) on Information Technology (IT) Expenditures" and "How to Formulate Your IT Strategy" respectively. I attended both presentations in rooms designed to hold 150 to 200. But in both there were fewer than a dozen people, including me. Both sessions were well presented in lay terminology that, it seemed to me, any businessperson could easily follow.

Why then, at the largest annual conference for mainstream healthcare executives (attended by over 4,400 that year), were two sessions on incredibly important yet commonly misunderstood topics so dismally attended? Both John and Rick are well known and have been leaders in the CIO ranks for decades. I looked for other competing sessions/topics opposite their respective timeslots on the agenda but found no obvious draws that could have kept attendees away from these sessions.

I reflected on my experiences with executives I have worked for and with, over the course of my career. It seemed to me that for many of these executives, managing IT was a magical craft. They did not necessarily want to know how it worked; they just wanted a "Merlin" for a CIO to magically "make it all work." But why, then, for two topics such as these, presented by two of the luminaries in the field of healthcare IT, would very few of the thousands of healthcare executives at the 2003 ACHE Congress attend presentations on topics that should have been of interest to them?

The mystery continues. During that same 2003 ACHE Congress I visited the Health Administration Press book fair that was set up in the exhibit area. There were literally hundreds of texts on all kinds of subjects from negotiating, to ethics, to healthcare finance and the like. But there were only two texts on healthcare IT! I was stunned. Information is the lifeblood of healthcare organizations. It is typically underutilized (translate to strategic opportunity), and yet the infrastructure (the heart, veins and arteries, if you will) of information is information technology. The effective use and management of IT have consistently been cited by the press as critically important in every industry for over 30 years and in healthcare for the past 15 years (marked by the awakening sound heralded by the Institute of Medicine's seminal 1991 publication, *The Computer-Based Patient Record*[1]). In the decade that followed, federal regulators took notice of the lack of action in leveraging IT in healthcare and set off a virtual avalanche of federal legislation and structures designed to get the healthcare industry to take IT-related action (e.g., HIPAA, Medical Error Act, Medication Error Act, establishing a National Coordinator for Healthcare IT in the Department of Health and Human Services). So again, why the lack of interest from the attendees?

It dawned on me that, while a CEO may not want to participate in auditor-level presentations on Sarbanes-Oxley (he or she has a CFO "partner" for that), the CEO would want to attend presentations that covered the high level implications of Sarbanes-Oxley and to gain counsel on the kinds of things he or she should be doing to ensure adequate oversight of the enterprise's financial activities. Similarly, for IT-related content, the challenge was presenting the material in a way that would compel the CEO's interest and to communicate the message that truly leveraging IT and harnessing its value was a partnership between, ultimately, the CEO and the CIO.

This book represents our attempt to both demystify the big topics in IT management for mainstream healthcare executives, such as CEOs, COOs, CFOs, CMOs, and CNOs, as well as to provide a reference source for CIOs as they work with their executive peers to better leverage IT in their respective organizations. We have attempted to assemble both CEO and CIO authors from across the spectrum of the healthcare industry—to present both perspectives, if you will, on this essential partnership. The terminology is intended for maximum understanding by non-IT folks.

The book begins with a prologue of a fictitious CEO, Sam Weatherspoon, as he starts his day at a fictitious healthcare organization, Ingalls Community Hospital. Each chapter attempts to help Sam, our fictitious CEO, demystify IT and implement best practices in IT management and oversight. With chapter titles such as "Where's the Beef: Getting Value from Your IT Investments" and "Outsourcing and the Merits of Marriage" and chapter content that is primarily intended for a non-IT audience, we hope the book resonates with the entire "C-suite" of executives. With increased pressure from all fronts (legislators, regulators, employers and consumers), we prescribe a healthy dose of partnering to harness the promised value of the significant investments that will be made in IT over the coming years. We hope this text provides some insight into ways to begin, sustain or enhance that essential partnership between the CEO and the CIO. Happy reading.

Detlev H. (Herb) Smaltz

1. Dick R, Steen E (eds): *The Computer-Based Patient Record: An Essential Technology for Health Care.* Washington DC: Institute of Medicine, National Academy Press; 1991.

Prologue

John P. Glaser, PhD, FCHIME, FHIMSS

Sam Weatherspoon, the Chief Executive Officer (CEO) of Ingalls Community Hospital, leaned back in his chair and gazed out his office window at the city lights.

Another long day, culminating in a dinner meeting with a group of restless physicians.

He replayed the events of the day. Did we make any progress? Were new problems identified? What do I need to follow up on tomorrow?

As he reflected on the day, the number of discussions and issues that focused on information technology (IT) struck him. Too many times IT featured prominently in the conversations—and not in a positive way.

CHAPTER 1: IT GOVERNANCE

At their breakfast meeting to discuss next year's budget, the Chief Financial Officer (CFO) reviewed the requests for IT capital. Just like last year, the requests dwarfed the capital targeted for IT projects. The CFO angrily commented on the insatiable appetite for IT, the cost of IT and the disorganized approach that Ingalls had to reviewing and prioritizing its IT demands. There had to be a more rational way to set the IT agenda.

The CFO went on to complain about an IT revenue cycle project. Finance and IT had disagreements about which vendor to pick. Finance liked the features and capabilities of Vendor A. IT liked Vendor B's technology. Finance and IT were at a stalemate. It was not clear who had the authority to pick the vendor and on what basis the vendor should be selected.

CHAPTER 2: WIREHEADS AND TECHNOPHOBES

Sam's meeting with the Chief Nursing Officer (CNO) had her grumbling about the wireless medication administration project. The IT team kept talking a foreign language, throwing out terms such as clamshells, LEAP, and robustness of network failover. She didn't understand any of it nor why she should need to do so.

1

She did want to know whether wireless would work or not. Were there any constraints in the technology that would hinder use by the nurses? How expensive was the technology?

     Her questions went unanswered.

CHAPTER 3: ART OF BUSINESS AND IT STRATEGIC ALIGNMENT

One of the trustees called to discuss a strategic planning meeting that had occurred the week before. The meeting had focused on a range of issues confronting Ingalls: lowering the costs of operations, addressing a nursing shortage and morale issues, and developing an outpatient strategy in the southern suburbs.

     The trustee, the CEO of a local bank, had commented on his organization's strategy development process. He noted how important IT was to their ability to execute their strategy. He asked Sam about the IT implications of the Ingalls strategy.

     Sam frowned and answered that he didn't know. IT was certainly busy and was spending a lot of money, but it was not clear to him that those efforts were advancing the strategy.

CHAPTER 4: GETTING VALUE FROM YOUR IT INVESTMENTS

A meeting to prepare for the budget retreat had focused on criteria for selecting capital projects. Operating margins were going to be tight again and the amount of available new capital was going to be smaller than Sam would like.

     Sam thought that the criteria proposed were reasonable: improving patient safety, increasing revenue, decreasing costs, improving service and enhancing quality of care. But he worried about the leadership team's ability to compare proposals that led to different value propositions. How do you compare an investment that improves patient safety with one that reduces costs? This was going to be particularly challenging for the IT project proposals that seemed to have a preponderance of "softer outcome" value propositions.

     Sam was not pleased by his realization that even the prior years' investments in IT projects, which claimed high significant cost reduction or revenue enhancement outcomes, had not seemed to have resulted in any significant margin improvement.

     Where did the gains go?

CHAPTER 5: ASSESSING YOUR IT ORGANIZATION'S PERFORMANCE

During a hallway conversation, the Chief Medical Officer (CMO) took the opportunity to complain about the time it took IT to implement systems. And the physicians viewed the systems that were delivered as decidedly mediocre. Moreover, the CMO had been to a conference last week and heard a talk from a CIO on the east coast about an incredible set of applications that had been implemented over what seemed to be an amazingly short period of time.

     Why can't our IT group do what the speaker's organization appeared to have done?

     Sam was not sure how to respond. His previous discussions with the Ingalls Chief Information Officer (CIO) had led him to be quite empathetic to the difficulty of implementing complex applications and the challenges of dealing with vendors. Nonetheless, was the Ingalls IT group mediocre at best?

CHAPTER 6: OUTSOURCING AND THE MERITS OF MARRIAGE

While hurrying through lunch at his desk, Sam scanned the Wall Street Journal. He took the time to read an article on IT outsourcing. The article featured several Fortune 100 companies that had moved large portions of information services (IS) overseas and had achieved significant reductions in IT costs (some in excess of 30%) and had improved the quality of IT services.

It sounded almost too good to be true. The Ingalls experiences in outsourcing dietary and security were not regarded as successes, and perhaps outsourcing IT would be a similarly mixed experience. But the companies mentioned in the article were good companies run by presumably very capable managers.

CHAPTER 7: THE CEO-CIO RELATIONSHIP

During his quarterly meeting with the CIO, Sam discussed the CIO's recent annual performance review. The CIO, while having had several significant accomplishments, had clearly struggled in other areas.

The IT group had not been as effective as hoped in helping the organization advance its efforts to improve access. The new scheduling system project was over budget and took much longer than planned to implement. The CIO, trying not to be too defensive, had responded that the access plans were muddled and the committee overseeing the changes could not make up its mind on several issues.

Sam noted that the managers of the pharmacy were complaining that the implementation of their new system had not resulted in the hoped-for improvements in pharmacy services. The CIO retorted that pharmacy had to exert leadership in revamping their processes. IT could not do it for them.

Sam also commented on the growth in the IT budget—a growth that every year was much larger than the growth in the overall organization's budget. If this trend kept going, IT was going to erase the already too-thin operating margin. The CIO complained about the constant tidal wave of new requests for IT services and applications and the "heroic" IT efforts to respond to it all.

At times during the discussion, Sam wondered if the two of them worked for the same organization and interacted with the same people.

CHAPTER 8: BUILDING A KNOWLEDGE-ENABLED ORGANIZATION

During Sam's meeting with the Chief Operating Officer (COO), they reviewed their efforts to improve the operating margin. The COO commented that they still could not get good data on costs and revenue by clinical service line or by physician. In addition, a myriad of issues plagued their efforts to improve the revenue cycle. The two major reasons that claims wound up in the error queue were the lack of a diagnosis on orders and missing documentation to support the claim.

Sam wondered why they had these problems since they had recently implemented an integrated suite of clinical and financial applications. The COO noted that the suite should have corrected these issues.

When Sam asked why they seemed to have mountains of data but not enough information, the COO was at a loss to explain.

CHAPTER 9: TO CENTRALIZE OR DECENTRALIZE?

Sam believed that he was a pretty smart guy. He had done well in school and was sure that a large part of this success had to do with his being very intelligent and having good management instincts.

However, he felt lost when the CIO (and now even some of physicians and his staff) talked about the technical aspects of IT. And perhaps because he found the jargon so confusing, Sam felt poorly equipped to hold a conversation on how to manage the networks, servers, and operating systems that formed the foundation of Ingalls' applications.

This unease with the topic went from annoying to concerning during the conversations that centered on the IT capital budget. Sam experienced similar concerns when he was asked to arbitrate a dispute between IT and some department that wanted to implement its own network or manage its own applications or pick a vendor that used "non-standard" technology.

Sam felt that he needed a glossary.

Tired from the day, Sam decided to head home, ignoring the pile of papers and e-mail that awaited his attention. Tomorrow he was going to have to begin to spend more time on the IT issues of Ingalls.

CHAPTER 1

Who's Minding the Store? Effective IT Governance

Walter E. Menning, FHIMSS, and Randy Carpenter, MSHI, CPHIMS

Sam Weatherspoon reflected on his numerous discussions of the previous day. The common thread of IT issues was something he felt committed to understand and to fix. Sam had no mistaken impressions about his being an expert in this area. That was precisely why he had created a Chief Information Officer (CIO) position several years ago.

Over the course of his career in healthcare Sam had experienced first hand the growth in use of computer technology. From the business office and back office administrative functions it seemed as though information systems had metastasized throughout the hospital and physicians' offices on campus. Increasingly, systems were being used to support clinical activity and patient care. He was grateful that he had sidestepped more than a decade of disappointment from the hype and overheated rhetoric of healthcare IS vendors. It was now clear that IT had become an integral component in the delivery of quality healthcare.

As his own organization had grown through acquisitions and management contracts, he learned the difficulty of sharing information between and among incompatible and disparate systems within his extended organization. These barriers, combined with an endless stream of regulatory changes, presented Sam and his senior management with requests that resulted in an ever increasing IT budget.

Sam decided to involve his CIO in finding a solution for his organization. Here is how their conversation started:

"(CIO), I am convinced we need to review the way our organization makes decisions about information technology. Before we form another committee or task force I think each of us should do some homework. I intend to speak with some of my colleagues around the country to learn how they approach decision making about information systems. What type of structure do they use? Who are the key players involved? How are capital budgets determined and major projects funded? Do they have a set of processes or procedures that are used consistently? Are there lessons they have learned that they are willing to share with us?

"I suggest that you contact some of your counterparts as well and ask a similar set of questions. While you're at it, you should attempt to find out about the role that your fellow

CIOs play in the decision making within their respective organizations. Let's compare notes in a couple weeks to see what we have learned. Let me know how I can help."

Almost a month had elapsed when Sam sat down with the CIO to review what they had learned. They both had been successful in contacting what they considered to be a reasonable cross section of healthcare organizations. A summary of what they learned about the various structures used to govern IT follows.

ALTERNATIVE MODELS OF IT GOVERNANCE: CURRENT PRACTICES IN HEALTHCARE

Executive Council

A model based on an executive council includes the senior executives within the healthcare organization (CEO, CFO, CMO, CIO, hospital administrator and other senior executives). The council may designate specific meetings of its membership to focus on information system-related topics or it may integrate information systems (IS) discussions as a part of the regular business agenda. The CEO typically chairs these meetings. Within larger healthcare organizations and integrated delivery systems, the full enterprise is the focus of the discussion and decisions. Individual hospitals and clinics may have their own council or oversight committee to address 'local' needs and issues. The frequency of meetings devoted to IS varies among the organizations using this model. Bimonthly or quarterly meetings seem to be the most popular.

IS Executive Steering Committee

This model includes a subset of the organization's senior executives combined with major stakeholders or users of IS resources. As is the case with the executive council, the steering committee focuses on strategy, policy and project proposals with broad organizational impact. (A more complete discussion of committee roles and responsibilities is included in the following section entitled **Major Roles of IT Governance**.) The chair of this committee is likely to be the CEO or a physician executive. In an academic medical center there is active participation by key representatives of research and education. The frequency of meetings of the steering committee is usually monthly. Subcommittees or task forces are appointed to address specific functions or processes such as information security or digital imaging.

Clinical Systems Oversight Committee

Another model in use is a committee structure that focuses on clinical applications. This may be due to the greatly increased emphasis that has been placed on clinical systems in recent years. This model has involvement of a broad cross section of physicians and is chaired by a physician. The agenda of this committee often seeks to improve patient safety and to gain acceptance and increased use of clinical systems such as computerized provider order entry (CPOE) by the full medical staff. Oversight committees meet monthly or bimonthly.

IS Advisory Committee

A somewhat "softer" model of governance is the advisory model. Committee membership includes a broad variety of stakeholders with an interest in the organization's utilization of IT. The CIO frequently chairs such a committee. Advisory committees frequently originate as a search committee appointed to interview and select a new CIO. The committee continues to meet with the new executive after he or she joins the organization. Alternatively, the advisory group may be formed early in the tenure of the new CIO. Input and advice is provided on a wide variety of topics. Agendas are flexible and meetings tend to have greater informality. It is not uncommon for the advisory committee to evolve into a more formal, structured oversight forum.

Ad Hoc (or None)

Many healthcare organizations do not have a formal structure for IT governance. Neither Sam nor his CIO was able to completely determine how the major IT-related decisions were made in these situations. Very likely a close relationship between the CEO and CIO resulted in the decisions as needed. The executive leadership team may be convened or consulted periodically as needed.

MAJOR ROLES OF IT GOVERNANCE

There is a strong pattern in the roles played by IT governance committees. The following discussion describes the major roles—those that recurred in multiple interviews. Note that numerous variations in the use of these roles exist. It is highly unlikely that all of these roles appear in the charter of the IT governance committee of a single organization. The organizations that Sam and his CIO talked to used the roles identified in combinations that merit further study.[1]

Strategy

Most prevalent in the discussion of IT governance was consideration of the healthcare organization's IT strategy. In almost every instance this meant that the IT governance structure sponsored the IT strategic planning process and the resulting plan.

Formulating the strategy involved committee members embracing a "big picture" view of capabilities across the entire enterprise. Parochial interests are put aside or put into perspective with the larger needs of the organization. Updating and refreshing the IT strategic plan are part of the continuing responsibility of the governance body.

Alignment

The enterprise perspective extends to support the alignment of the IT strategy with the overall organization's strategy. Process improvement or process redesign initiatives across the organization are integrated with appropriate IT initiatives. Similarly, programs to address patient safety or quality of care are aligned with requisite IT resources and systems.

IT Infrastructure

As the investment in and deployment of IT has grown rapidly over the past decade, IT governance has increasingly focused on modernizing and upgrading its underlying infrastructure. Local and wide area networks, highly available computing resources and help desk support are examples of centrally managed assets needed for the delivery of patient care and efficient operation of a current day medical center. IT governance is positioned to survey the organization-wide demand for capital expenditures and to determine a capital budget to maintain and grow the IT infrastructure.

IT Architecture and Standards
A corollary to determining appropriate allocation of IT capital spending is establishing the policies and rules used regarding the organization's data, technology and applications. The role of governance is to provide oversight to the creation and implementation of these policies and to understand the longer-term effects of adopting a new technology as well as the need to sunset older technologies.

Setting Priorities
Another role frequently performed by the IT steering committee is that of ranking priorities for projects, initiatives or requests that arise during a planning cycle. These may be initiatives that are not specifically identified in the IT strategic plan.

Policies and Principles
The oversight group may also be involved in setting and endorsing IT-related policies that are administered across the healthcare organization. Examples include policies related to information security, internal charging for IT services, archiving and record retention and Internet access.

Post-Implementation Reviews and Organizational Learning
There are numerous approaches used by IT governance to review major projects at various stages of implementation. A particularly important milestone occurs when implementation is completed. Assessment measures include the traditional measure of "on time and on budget" as well as assessment of return on investment and the achievement of objectives and benefits outlined in the original project proposal. There is an opportunity to share lessons learned during the project life cycle with other initiatives in earlier project phases.

Other Observations
Sam and his CIO learned that other organizations they had spoken with had IT committees that had been in place for long periods of time. Several of the people they interviewed had formed committees that had been operating successfully for 10 to 15 years. When Sam sat down with his CIO the stories they shared were quite positive and contained many helpful suggestions.

IT GOVERNANCE IN OTHER INDUSTRIES
At this point it is appropriate to review a major research study on IT governance outside of healthcare that has taken place over the past several years. The study was performed at the MIT Sloan School of Management, Center for Information Systems Research; it reviewed IT governance of more than 250 companies in 23 countries. The companies involved in the study represent a broad cross section of industries. One of the major conclusions is that while top-performing enterprises governed IT with different models, they were consistently successful in obtaining value from IT where

others failed. It is estimated that the top-performing companies produced up to 40% greater return than their competitors for the same IT investment by implementing effective IT governance.[2]

The study provides a number of observations that may prove useful to the CEO and CIO of larger healthcare organizations and integrated delivery systems as they contemplate the appropriate IT governance structure for their organizations.

IT Principles Decisions High-Level Statements about How IT Is Used in the Business		
IT Architecture Decisions Organizing logic for data, applications, and infrastructure captured in a set of policies, relationships, and technical choices to achieve desired business and technical standardization and integration	**IT Infrastructure Decisions** Centrally coordinated, shared IT services that provide the foundation for the enterprise's IT capability	**IT Investment and Prioritization Decisions** Decisions about how much and where to invest in IT, including project approvals and justification techniques
	Business Applications Needs Specifying the business need for purchased or internally developed IT applications	

Figure 1-1. Key IT Governance Decisions[3]

For example, Figure 1-1 depicts the major IT decision categories that need to be addressed: principles, architecture, infrastructure strategies, business application needs and investment and prioritization. Similarly, Figure 1-2 summarizes the IT governance archetypes, or models, identified during the study. These archetypes bare strong similarity to the models identified by Sam and his CIO, although healthcare organizations had no corresponding models for the "IT Monarchy" or the "IT Duopoly." They also identify who within the enterprise holds the decision rights and input rights for each governance model. The study uses decision rights to formulate a definition of IT governance: "Specifying the decision rights and accountability framework to encourage desirable behavior in the use of IT."[4]

The study concludes that effective IT governance is the single most important predictor of the value an organization generates from IT.

IT Governance Archetypes				
Decision rights or inputs for a particular IT decision are held by:		CxO Level Execs	Corp. IT and/or Business Unit IT	Business Unit Leaders or Process Owners
Business Monarchy	A group of, or individuals, business executives (i.e., CxOs). Includes committees comprised of senior business executives (may include CIO). Excludes IT executives acting independently.	✓		
IT Monarchy	Individuals or groups of IT executives		✓	
Feudal	Business unit leaders, key process owners or their delegates			✓
Federal	C-level executives and at least one other business group (e.g., CxO and BU leaders)— IT executives may be additional participants. Equivalent to a country and its states working together.	✓	✓	✓
		✓		✓
IT Duopoly	IT executives and one other group (e.g., CxO or BU leaders)	✓	✓	
			✓	✓
Anarchy	Each individual user			

Figure 1-2. IT Governance Archetypes[5]

EVOLUTION AND MATURITY OF IT GOVERNANCE

Determining which governance model fits appropriately within an organization also aligns directly with where the organization is from an IT maturity model perspective. As indicated in Figure 1-3 there are several levels where an organization's IT role may fit. For many organizations IT is primarily a service provider, yet IT strives to become more of a business enabler enroute to fulfilling some level of strategic partnership. Evolving from a service provider to a business enabler role fits well with solid IT governance processes and allows the IT function to focus on the medium to long-term view.

For most organizations that fit in the service provider role with their IT function, it could take several years to mature the IT model to align with an evolving governance structure and reach the ultimate goal of a sound strategic partnership.

GETTING STARTED: WHAT WORKS

Sam decided it would be best for his organization to form an IT Steering Committee. He tested the idea with his executive and clinical leadership to gain feedback and determine interest among individuals within this group. This worked well because several members of the executive team felt over-extended while several others expressed a keen interest in being involved in IT oversight. Sam and his CIO met to develop a start-up strategy, which included six main components:

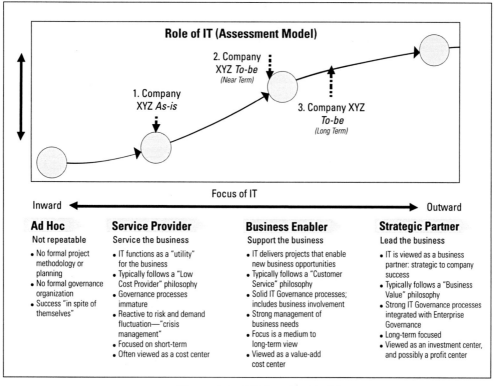

Figure 1-3. IT Maturity Model

1. **Committee Charter.** A draft charge for the IT Steering Committee was developed to share with prospective members and for discussion at the committee's kick off meeting. The draft charter is shown in Figure 1-4.

2. **Membership.** Strike a healthy balance of senior administrative and clinical leadership. Avoid starting with too large a membership. This has the potential of bogging down early discussion and deliberations. It is better to add people over time than to ask people to withdraw from the committee.

3. **Set Expectations for Committee Members.** During the early phases there can be significant time commitments. Regular attendance and participation are important to the success of the governance activity. Expectations about the term of service on the committee should also be made explicit. While some members serve by virtue of their position within the organization, many stakeholders may serve variable terms. The effort to orient new members should not be underestimated. A term of four years or more should be sought to ensure continuity in the deliberations of the committee.

4. **Follow the Basics of Conducting Effective Meetings.** The rules for effective meetings apply to IT governance just as they do in other organizational matters. A well-planned agenda with appropriate reference material distributed well in advance of the meeting are the first order of business. Well-prepared presentation material and sufficient time allocated for discussion will help the committee accomplish its purpose.

**Ingalls Hospital
Information Systems Executive Steering Committee
Charge and Membership**

<u>**Members:**</u>

Chief Executive Officer, Chair
Vice President for Medical Affairs
Vice President for Financial Affairs
Vice President – Operations
Vice President – Nursing
Vice President – Human Resources
Medical Director of Laboratory Services
Vice President – Health System Affiliates
Chief Information Officer, Secretary

<u>**Charge:**</u>

❑ **Direction Setting**
   Review and concur with major IT initiatives; ensure that Information Systems Strategic Plan is aligned with Ingalls Hospital's overall business plans and goals.

❑ **Prioritization**
   Evaluate major proposals and determine organizational IT priorities based on support for strategic goals and business initiatives.

❑ **Budget Approval and Resource Allocation**
   Establish an adequate funding level to accomplish approved projects. Funding decisions will address staffing levels and appropriation of capital for IT infrastructure.

❑ **Project Management**
   Evaluate performance against committed milestones. Sponsor post-implementation assessment of financial impact, benefits and lessons learned.

❑ **Policy Development**
   Oversee the development of policies and standards to ensure the effective and efficient utilization of organizational resources.

<u>**Meeting Schedule:**</u>
The Information Systems Executive Steering Committee will meet from 12:00 noon to 2:00 p.m. on the third Wednesday of each month in the Board Room.

Figure 1-4. Draft Charter, IT Steering Committee

5. **Delegate Effort as Needed.** It is not uncommon for recurring issues to arise during the course of normal governance committee business. When this happens, the committee should seek resolution of the issue(s) without bogging down the entire group. Some examples might be policies (or lack of policies) related to remote computer access, use and organizational support of personal digital assistants (PDAs), and standards and frequency of password changes.

When issues such as these consume unplanned time on the committee's agenda, consider appointing a workgroup or task force of people with the expertise and related experience to study the issue and propose a recommended solution. This approach has the benefit of keeping the committee focused on its mainstream role as well as involving others in understanding and resolving organization-wide issues. It is entirely possible for some of the workgroups to evolve into standing subcommittees of the IT governance committee.

6. **Educate Early and Often.** Creating a common foundation and frame of reference among the oversight committee members will be important to the committee's start up and continued success. Depending on the seniority and experience of members, education on the role and nature of governance may be an appropriate early topic. Tours of key information infrastructure areas, high-level demonstrations of systems in use and high-level coverage of material will aid in demystifying subject matter under discussion.

PITFALLS AND ITEMS TO AVOID

The realm of IT governance has great potential for differences of opinion on resource allocation, priorities, technical direction and solution sets chosen. Many of the possible emotional disagreements can be avoided if members keep in mind the true role of governance. The focus of discussion should be on the "What," not the "How" in setting overall direction and strategy for IT across the enterprise. This becomes much less of an issue as members become accustomed to their roles and to working with each other. This is particularly true of the first several pitfalls discussed in this section.

Micromanagement

The members of a steering committee or governance council should avoid the inclination to supervise or "dive into the weeds" regarding the functioning of the IT organizational units. Dialog should occur regarding the ends, or objectives, and not the means, or procedures, in use within IT. For example, while an individual member may have a deeply seated desire to know why Company XYZ was selected as the supplier for desktop computers, the discussion that follows is highly likely to divert the full committee from its focus. A preferred way to frame the question would be to ask: "What is the process used to select suppliers of equipment such as desktop computers?" Even better would be a discussion of the total cost of ownership of desktop computers, upgrade and replacement policies and the role of desktop computers in the organization's information architecture.

Personal or Local Agendas

It is extremely important that all committee members put on their governance "hats" and put aside departmental or personal issues as the committee conducts its business. Again, this behavior diverts the full committee from its purpose and should be redirected to an appropriate one-on-one discussion at another time and setting.

"Technospeak"

The language of governance should be the language of healthcare business. There will be numerous times when the CIO or various members of the CIO's management team will be asked to brief the committee on specific projects, aspects of IT infrastructure or architecture. All too frequently the acronyms and jargon unique to IT creep into a briefing, eyes glaze over and the true message is lost in technobabble. The CIO should use this opportunity to coach his or her staff on a higher-level approach to presenting material for the governance group. If necessary, the material to be covered should be rehearsed to ensure straightforward and understandable treatment of discussion items.

Under-Delegation

Failure to deal with recurring issues by appointing task forces or work groups as described earlier in this chapter can cause the committee to bog down and divert its attention in counter-productive ways.

CONCLUSIONS

At the conclusion of the inaugural IT Steering Committee meeting, Sam invited his CIO back to his office to debrief on the discussions that took place and to plan some next steps. Sam was quite pleased with the outcome of the first meeting. Yes, there were some animated discussions, but even these served to highlight the need to revisit many of these topics to educate members and to clarify several misperceptions that surfaced. He and the CIO identified topics likely to span the next five or six meetings. He asked the CIO to begin to put together material for discussions on an overview of major vendors used at Sam's organization, Ingalls, on the topics of wireless technology, the overall IT budget, and the current portfolio of clinical applications.

The dialog that began that day will serve Sam and his organization well. The executive team under Sam's leadership demonstrated a factor critical to the success of IT governance: executive commitment. Collectively their commitment to governance will help demystify IT and help others understand how decisions related to IT are made. Ultimately they will create a climate that encourages desirable behavior in the use of IT and the value this use of IT generates for the organization.

An equally important success factor to executive commitment is the open dialog and communication promoted by the IT governance process. This extends beyond the communication within the IT Steering Committee and its visitors. Sharing of information of the decisions and proceedings of the governance structure helps to address the communications gap between IT fact and fiction frequently evidenced in healthcare organizations. This becomes an important element in bridging the communication gap that is discussed in Chapter 2.

Walter E. Menning, FHIMSS, is the Vice Chair of Information Services at the Mayo Clinic in Rochester, Minnesota. Mr. Menning is a Fellow in the Healthcare Information and Management Systems Society (HIMSS), where he served as a member of the Board of Directors from 1998–2002 and Board Chairman from 2000–2001. He is the 1997 recipient of the John E. Gall Jr. CIO Award for outstanding contributions to the field of healthcare information technology management.

Randy Carpenter, MSHI, CPHIMS, is Senior Vice President and Chief Information Officer for HealthSouth Corporation. He has over 25 years experience in various information technology management capacities and is currently a member of both the Healthcare Information Management Systems Society (HIMSS) and the College of Healthcare Information Management Executives (CHIME).

References

1. The material included in Alternative Models and Major Roles of IT Governance is based upon a survey of members of the Healthcare Information Systems Executive Association (HISEA) conducted during the period August 27–September 25, 2004. The authors wish to express their appreciation to members of HISEA who participated in this effort.
2. Weill P, Ross JW: *IT Governance: How Top Performers Manage IT Decision Rights for Superior Results.* Boston, MA: Harvard Business School Press; 2004.
3. Weill P, Ross JW: *IT Governance: How Top Performers Manage IT Decision Rights for Superior Results.* Boston, MA: Harvard Business School Press; 2004; p 27.
4. Weill P, Ross JW: *IT Governance: How Top Performers Manage IT Decision Rights for Superior Results.* Boston, MA: Harvard Business School Press; 2004; p 8.
5. Weill P: Don't Just Lead, Govern: How Top-Performing Firms Govern IT, *Massachusetts Institute of Technology or MIS Quarterly Executive.* March 2004; 3(1): 5.

Bibliography

Bell M: *Leading and Managing in the Virtual Matrix Organization.* Gartner, Inc., March 11, 2004.

Bowen TS: The Right Way to Steer IT, *CIO Magazine.* September 1, 2004.

Bowen TS: If It Ain't Broke, Why Assign a Committee to Fix It? *CIO Magazine.* September 1, 2004.

Dallas S: *Business Management of IT: Organization and Governance.* Gartner, Inc.

Dallas S: *Six IT Governance Rules to Boost IT and User Credibility.* Gartner, Inc., October 9, 2002.

Dallas S: *IT Governance Requires Decision-Making Guidelines.* Gartner, Inc., January 19, 2004.

Dallas S: *CIO Update: IT Governance Rules to Boost IS Organization and Business Unit Credibility.* Gartner, Inc., December 4, 2002.

Dallas S, Bell M: *The Need for IT Governance: Now More Than Ever.* Gartner, Inc., January 20, 2004.

Dragoon A: Deciding Factors, *CIO Magazine.* April 15, 2003.

Dreyfuss C: *Create a Governance Architecture That Adapts to Change.* Gartner, Inc., November 26, 2003.

Gerrard M: *Creating an Effective IT Governance Process.* Gartner, Inc., November 20, 2003.

Light M: *Project Offices Are Key Components of IT Governance.* Gartner, Inc., November 17, 2003.

Mingay S, Bittinger S: *Combine CobiT and ITIL for Powerful IT Governance.* Gartner, Inc., June 10, 2003.

Morello D, Bell M, Dallas S: *Demystifying IT Governance.* Gartner, Inc., January 20, 2004.

Neela MA, Mahoney J: *Work With, Not Against, Your Culture to Refine IT Governance.* Gartner, Inc., November 13, 2003.

Roberts J: *Delivering Business Value through Effective Governance.* Gartner, Inc., October 23, 2003.

Smith HA: *Advanced Practices in IT Structure and Governance Part I: Introduction and Conceptual Framework.* Queen's University, 2000–2002.

Smith HA: *IT Structure and Governance Part II: Principles, Guidelines and Trends.* Queen's University, 2000–2002.

Weill P: *Don't Just Lead, Govern: How Top-Performing Firms Govern IT,* Massachusetts Institute of Technology or MIS Quarterly Executive. March 2004, 3(1).

Weill P: *Don't Just Lead, Govern! Governing IT for Different Performance Goals,* Society of Information Management Academic Workshop. December, 2003.

Weill P, Ross JW: *IT Governance: How Top Performers Manage IT Decision Rights for Superior Results.* Boston MA, Harvard Business School Press; 2004.

Weill P, Woodham R: *Don't Just Lead, Govern: Implementing Effective IT Governance.* Massachusetts Institute of Technology; April 2002.

Wilkoff N: *Governing IT in the Enterprise.* Forrester Research, Inc.; July 30, 2004.

CHAPTER 2

Wireheads and Technophobes: Bridging the Communication Gap

Detlev H. (Herb) Smaltz, PhD, FHIMSS, CHE, CKM

Sam Weatherspoon's meeting with the Chief Nursing Officer (CNO) had her grumbling about the wireless medication administration project. The IS team kept talking a foreign language, throwing out terms such as clamshells, LEAP and robustness of network failover. She didn't understand any of it nor why she should need to do so.

She did want to know whether wireless would work or not. Were there any constraints in the technology that would hinder use by the nurses? How expensive was the technology?

Her questions went unanswered.

Both the academic [1,2,3] and mainstream[4] literature are full of studies and stories that lament the IT community's inability to communicate in terms that the business side of the house can understand. While the prescriptions for bridging the communication division between IT and the rest of the organization seem so obvious, few healthcare organizations are actually employing many of the means available to them to do so. A recent internal IT audit report from a major academic medical center cited lack of adequate communication about the IT agenda as one of the major discrepancy findings. The CIO of this organization later articulated numerous examples of how he felt he had communicated the IT agenda at every forum available to him. Yet the clinical department chairs who had overseen the audit perceived just the opposite in their audit findings.

The lack of common understanding about how IT can be used to achieve key organizational strategic objectives is at least one of the fundamental reasons that many organizations are not able to fully achieve their strategic visions. While some executives find it easy to blame the CIO for not making a better case for strategic IT projects in terms understandable by the top management team, common understanding is a two-way street. Figure 2-1 summarizes some of the complaints that CEOs and CIOs have about each other.

Complaints That CEOs Make about CIOs	Complaints That CIOs Make about CEOs
Communicate in technical terms instead of business terms	Are not comfortable sharing strategic objectives
Lose sight of the business when dealing with technological decisions	Resist having the CIO as a direct report or on the senior executive management team
Remain ignorant of the organization's customers and their needs	Refuse to explore how technology could solve business problems
Fail to protect the CEO from IT vendors	Persist in thinking about IT only for automating accounting functions
Obstructionists rather than enablers	Treat IT professionals as less than equals
Harbor judgments that non-technical people, such as most CEOs, are pitiful	Are too insecure to ask technical questions for fear of appearing ignorant

Figure 2-1. Sources of the IT Communications Gap[5]

As technology permeates almost every aspect of business and personal lives, it is important for both the CIO and the other executives in the organization to find ways to mutually bridge the communication gap that has been cited as dogging the CEO-CIO relationship for over at least the past decade.[6, 7, 8, 9, 10]

This chapter suggests actions that CEOs can take to mentor CIOs to communicate a clear, understandable message about IT and IT's potential to executives who may have quite varying degrees of general knowledge about technical issues. Additionally, it provides insight into organizational phenomena that suggest that communication skills are a prerequisite to building trusting relationships and acceptance as an executive peer. Finally, this chapter suggests ways CIOs can help their CEOs and other top executives in overcoming their fear and loathing of technology discussions via effective organizational communication mechanisms.

INDIVIDUAL LEVEL COMMUNICATIONS: TECHNOBABBLE VS. LAYPERSON'S LANGUAGE

Think for a moment about traveling to a foreign country—one in which English is not the common language. To prepare for the journey, some travelers take a crash course in an attempt to attain a conversational level in the second language. Others purchase one of those tiny translation books that can be referenced while abroad. But the reality is that those who have attempted either of the above quickly come to realize that, unless they have a phenomenal ability to quickly master foreign languages, neither approach works very well in helping to communicate with the residents of the foreign country in real time. Fortunately for U.S. residents, most of the rest of the world can speak English at an understandable level, quickly coming to the rescue with a courteous, friendly, "Can I help you; I speak English" when one makes a feeble attempt to speak their language.

There is a lesson to be learned here. While many arguments lament C-level executives (CEO, COO, CFO, CMO, CNO, and the like) for not applying themselves more to gaining an understanding of and appetite for learning how technology can leverage and/or transform their organizations, the reality is that technological advances are moving at break-neck speed and, by the way, the C-level executives continue to have their main jobs to deal with. So the author's bias is that CIOs should attempt to be more like citizens of foreign countries and learn to speak the English of C-level executives.

Ironically, CIOs who have come up through the technical ranks and are not formal members of the top executive management team or committee may not have had the exposure necessary to have learned to communicate in anything other than technobabble. So what can CEOs and the other members of the top management team do to mentor CIOs to bridge the communication gap that may exist between them? The author's own research in CIO effectiveness found that more important than reporting relationship is whether or not the CIO is a formal member of the organization's top management team.[11] Making CIOs a member of the top management team accomplishes a number of important things:

1. It communicates to the other executives in the organization that the CIO is a true executive peer and like the other top management executives is expected to contribute not just in their particular specialty area, but in the full spectrum of dialog that top management teams engage in to solve problems and forge new directions.
2. Via this regular, cross-functional dialog, the CIO is exposed to, and immersed in, the language of C-level executives—both business and clinical speak. The importance of immersion cannot be understated. The best way to learn a new language is via full immersion.
3. It provides the CEO, or the CIO's reporting officer, opportunities to provide regular mentoring feedback. For instance, right after a discussion during which the CEO feels the CIO used far too much technical jargon, he or she can take the opportunity to discuss alternate ways that the CIO could have communicated the message for greater effectiveness. Over time, the CIO will learn to consistently articulate technical issues in a myriad of ways. For the CEO, COO, and CFO, this will be in business operational and fiscal terms, and for the CMO and CNO, it will be in operational and clinical terms.
4. Finally, it builds trusting relationships between the CIO and the other members of the top management team. Frankly, it is difficult to trust someone whom we cannot understand, or someone whom we have not had the opportunity to observe in their actions and reactions to various situations. Because most IT projects easily run in the millions and tens of millions of dollars, communication and hence trust are paramount. Constant interaction on the top management team is one way for CIOs to learn to communicate and build trust.

This author is not suggesting that simply by bringing a CIO into the top management team will the CIO be transformed into a lean, mean business-speaking C-level machine. There are some who simply will not feel comfortable at that level of the organization. Perhaps these individuals are better suited to the Chief Technology Officer (CTO) role and the organization might be better served with someone in the CIO position who is comfortable discussing and engaging in cross-functional business and clinical issues. However, a CEO does the organization a great disservice and most likely decreases the impact that IT could potentially have in an organization if the CIO is not formally placed on the organization's top executive management team.

INDIVIDUAL LEVEL COMMUNICATIONS: MENTORING "WIREHEAD" CIOS

CEOs can mentor CIOs to follow some obvious, and perhaps not so obvious, practices to better communicate with the other top management executives in the organization. These include the following:

1. Refrain from using technical acronyms when speaking to the other top executives or line managers, even for phrases that the CIO may think are in the common vernacular. Spell out acronyms if there is even one person in the room who may not be familiar with it (e.g., not "WiFi" but "wireless"; not "VoIP" but "voice over IP," which is basically telephone communications using a pre-existing local area network instead of the phone company's lines).

2. Use appropriate analogies. Nothing provides a common frame of reference more effectively than do analogies. While these can be overused if not regularly updated (one CEO recently declared, "I'm going to strangle the next technical person who tries to use the 'railroad track gauge' analogy on me to try to sell me on rearchitecting our network infrastructure again"), they become powerful tools for understanding and discourse if carefully selected for the topic at hand. Analogies can readily be mined from daily transactions with clinicians and other business people within and outside the organization. For instance, as the Chief Knowledge Officer (CKO) for the Air Force Medical Service, one of the most useful clinical analogies for the topic of knowledge management came from this author's interactions with the Air Force Medical Service CIO, Dr. Janice Lee. She noted that the synergies and alignment that we were trying to gain by interconnecting the various functional "communities of practice" within the Air Force Medical Service was much like taking individual heart muscle cells, which beat independently of one another when separated but quickly synchronize and beat in unison when they are put into contact with one another. Apparently this is a principle taught in virtually all medical schools and therefore would serve well when trying to communicate to a clinical audience the impact that interconnecting functional communities of practice could have within an organization. Collect analogies from as many perspectives as possible and bring them to bear on pertinent technical topics to create a common frame of reference.

3. Network with the other executives. Get to know them beyond the boundaries of the organization. Play golf with them, go hiking, kayaking, shopping, skiing, or whatever common interests the parties have. Communicating in these more intimate settings creates obvious friendships and bonds of trust.

4. Learn to say "no" in a non-threatening way. The truth is that CIOs simply do not have the resources to accomplish every good project that comes from the myriad departments within your organization. Rather than saying "no" out of hand, establish a systematic process of getting to "yes" *for the appropriate projects*. CFOs have learned this well by adopting rigid "hurdle rate" criteria for weighing competing projects. CIOs should protect themselves by proactively ensuring that all IT projects go through the same acquisition approval process as other organizational investments. This is best done by selecting an appropriate governance model that covers organization-wide criteria for IT investments (see Chapter 1 on effective IT governance models, which cover this issue in depth).

ORGANIZATIONAL COMMUNICATIONS: THINGS CIOS CAN DO TO REDUCE TECHNOPHOBIA

While the CIO's interpersonal communication skills are important to effectively employing IT within organizations, equally important are IT-related organizational communication mechanisms discussed in the other chapters of this text (e.g., IT governance, IT performance measurement, and enterprise information management). It is this author's bias that within an organization it is virtually impossible to "over communicate" the IT agenda and how specific IT projects relate to the organization's overall strategic goals and objectives. Therefore, organizations that take the time to set up effective IT governance structures with enterprise-wide representation are, in a sense, "baking-in" processes that force cross-functional communication and increased understanding of the various IT initiatives that are going on at any given time.

However, IT governance is only one of the means with which to communicate the IT agenda and how it relates to, affects, and enhances the various business and clinical processes within the organization. Additional organizational IT communication mechanisms include, but are not limited to, the following suggestions.

Communicate via the main healthcare organization's media. CIOs need to ensure that they are proactively tasking internal resources to religiously provide relevant news about IT projects that are coming, status reports on current projects, and, finally, retrospective news to celebrate successes and inform how they positively affected operations. Employ all forms of media available such as organizational staff newsletters, patient-focused newsletters, the healthcare organization's main Web site, the IT organization's Web site, and the like. Most importantly, write in prose that is relevant and understandable to the intended audience. Again, it is virtually impossible to over-communicate the IT agenda.

Create palpable IT project future state visions. One extremely useful organizational communication mechanism is to create a palpable vision of a future state that truly resonates with the members of the entire healthcare organization, and then continually use this vision in all IT interdepartmental communications (as opposed to setting it on a shelf to collect dust).

To illustrate this, UAB Health System, at this writing, is embarking on a huge core clinical systems replacement effort. Working with Healthlink, the members of UAB's information services group and clinical departments created a vision statement of an optimal future state for UAB Health System's 1,000-bed academic acute care setting, University Hospital, as well as for its 470-physician ambulatory setting, the Kirklin Clinic (TKC). These vision documents and presentation slides (see Appendix 2-1 for an example of UAB's ambulatory optimal future state vision) are being used throughout the project to continually communicate the envisioned future state that will be enabled by the IT interventions, which are intentionally interwoven into the story and highlighted in boldface. These vision documents and slide presentations provide a consistent message about where UAB Health System wants to go and how IT specifically will help get it there, presented in a story-like fashion for ease of understanding. Additionally, UAB uses complementary presentation slides to drill down to ever increasing levels of granularity with respect to specific clinical and business workflow processes and how the envisioned IT interventions have the potential to positively affect them.

Finally, because the optimal future state story is about a fictitious character, Ralph, as he weaves his way through the healthcare enterprise, the project managers at UAB Health System use a manikin, complete with a "Ralph" ID badge. This is a creative way to constantly reinforce the vision in a way that exponentially stimulates conversation about, awareness of, and participation in the project.

If an IT project will affect more than one functional area (and almost all healthcare applications do), always develop a communication plan for the IT project. These IT project communication plans should always be co-developed with the main stakeholder/constituents of the project. For instance, the communication plan for a computer based provider order entry (CPOE) system should be codeveloped with whomever has been named the clinical project champion. If no one has been named (which is not ideal), then collaborate with some of the main physician users to develop the communication plan. This plan should cover topics such as developing the future state vision (see above) or the "formal messages" about the project and what its envisioned positive impacts will be; identifying potential media to communicate news about the project; and identifying individuals who can write news articles and develop a timeline/schedule for news releases and the like. Again, it is next to impossible to over-communicate the IT agenda. (See Appendix 2-2 for a sample IT project communication plan.)

Clearly define rules of engagement for IT-related acquisitions. The rules of engagement for IT-related acquisition processes should be clearly articulated in the organization's governance model (see Chapter 1 for a more in-depth discussion). Additionally, incentives should be in place to encourage following the governance model when acquiring functional IT as well as disincentives for departments that "go around the system." These rules of engagement embedded in governance structures and/or processes are really designed to openly communicate and vet the merits of various initiatives and, therefore, are incredibly useful in bridging the communication gap as IT projects are prioritized using the same criteria and vernacular as the other non-IT projects.

Even if not asked to do so by senior executive management, CIOs are encouraged to proactively put in place measurements and assessments of the IT organization's performance with respect to customer support responsiveness (help desk response times, time to resolution, satisfaction with help desk responsiveness) and impacts of each IT initiative (collect relevant baseline data prior to the project implementation and then collect "after" data to determine if envisioned benefits are realized). For a more in-depth discussion of IT organizational performance measurement, see Chapter 5.

The next time the senior executive team updates its strategic plan, consider developing a strategic data map in conjunction with the strategic plan as outlined in Chapter 8 of this text. More and more healthcare organizations are adopting strategic frameworks, such as Norton and Kaplan's Balanced Scorecard,[12] which demand additional work to identify measures of success for strategic plan initiatives. The activity of developing the strategic data map creates dialog that points to the strengths and weaknesses of organizational data in being able to assess strategic impact of various projects. This can spin off into a new effort to create better organizational level data capture strategies that benefit the organization as a whole in subsequent strategic planning sessions.

Consider setting up a technology assessment committee to proactively deal with what may clumsily be called "the tyranny of the conferences," or the "tyranny of the airplane magazines." The fact is that individuals from all over an organization get ideas all the time from conferences they attend or magazines they read that could potentially be breakthrough ideas for the organization. Technology assessment committees are designed to take ideas that include a technology component and quickly vet them for relevance, strategic impact, compatibility with existing infrastructure, and so forth. Again, such a forum creates opportunities for open dialog and communications that show that the IT department is being proactive rather than reactive.

Co-attend key professional conferences. If the American College of Healthcare Executives (ACHE) is the CEO's preferred professional association, have the CIO attend the next ACHE annual Congress on Healthcare Management with the CEO. If the Healthcare Information and Management Systems Society (HIMSS) is the CIO's preferred professional association, get the CEO to attend with the CIO. This co-attendance provides both executives with an opportunity to mentor one another about new advances and approaches in mainstream healthcare administration as well as healthcare IT and how they can be applied to the organization's strategic objectives.

These proactive steps create an open environment that facilitates dialog about IT and how IT can further the goals of the organization.

SUMMARY

As noted in the introduction, the prescriptions in this chapter seem incredibly obvious to this author and the editors of this book. The popular literature, however, suggests that these prescriptions are either not followed fully or have not generally been effective; therefore they are included in this text. This chapter is intended to complement the important communication mechanisms embedded in prescriptions from other chapters (Chapter 1 on IT governance, Chapter 5 on assessing IT performance, and Chapter 8 on building a knowledge-enabled organization).

There are a number of things that CEOs can do to mentor "wirehead" CIOs to become better communicators. CEOs who have not already done so can significantly increase the CIOs' communication skills over time (and ability to add value across the full range of organizational strategic objectives) via formal membership into the organization's senior executive management team/committee. For all major IT projects, CIOs are encouraged to develop, with the aid of key stakeholders, a relevant, palpable future vision state of how IT will enhance business and clinical processes and outcomes, and continually use this optimal future state vision in all communication avenues as the project is developed and implemented. Finally, CIOs are encouraged to develop a communications plan for IT projects and employ all available sources of media to communicate the IT agenda and how it relates to, affects, and enhances the organization's business and clinical processes. In healthcare organizations it is virtually impossible to over-communicate the IT agenda.

Detlev H. (Herb) Smaltz, PhD, FHIMSS, CHE, CKM, has a dual appointment at the University of Alabama at Birmingham (UAB) Health System, a $1 billion-plus academic center, where he is an Associate Professor in the Health Informatics Program and also *serves as the Chief Technology Officer. Prior to his appointment at UAB, Dr. Smaltz was the first-ever Chief Knowledge Officer for the Air Force Medical Service, a $6.2 billion globally distributed integrated delivery system. In previous positions, he served as the CIO for a 20-bed community hospital, a 301-bed academic medical center, a 5-state region, and a 7-country region. Dr. Smaltz is a Diplomate in the American College of Healthcare Executives and a Fellow in the Healthcare Information and Management Systems Society (HIMSS). He served on the HIMSS Board of Directors from 2002 to 2005 and as Vice-Chair of the same board from 2004 to 2005. He earned an MBA from the Ohio State University and a PhD from Florida State University.*

APPENDIX 2-1
UAB HEALTH SYSTEM'S OPTIMAL AMBULATORY FUTURE STATE

Ralph is a 65-year-old retired UAB employee. Ralph is thoroughly enjoying his new found free time and spends as much time at the beach as possible.

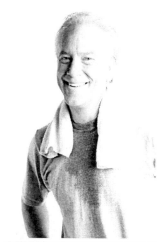

Ralph has always considered himself to be in excellent health—he rarely gets a cold, maintains good exercise and eating habits and makes sure he is seen annually by Dr. Smith, his internist at The Kirklin Clinic (TKC).

Lately, however, Ralph has noticed he has heartburn quite often and occasionally has also experienced some pain in his abdomen/chest. Ralph decides to make an appointment with Dr. Smith to get checked out.

Ralph obtains an appointment for the next day. He takes advantage of the option to access the **health information patient web portal** link. He successfully updates his past family, medical, social history and also types in his recent symptoms. From here he can also access patient education topics and even sees an area where he can post a confidential message to his physician.

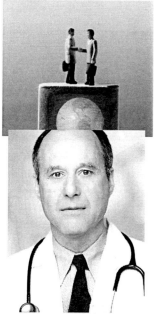

Later that same day at TKC, Ralph's physician, Dr. Smith, logs onto the ambulatory clinical system in his office to finish his records for that day. In the clinical system there is a **personal clinician view** that consolidates and displays a list of outstanding documents he needs to finish. He can also review multidisciplinary documentation, internal messages from colleagues and clinic staff. Dr. Smith has chosen to provide e-mail communication with his patients, which allows him to respond. This communication is managed through corporate guidelines and governance. From this area, he can also check his schedule for the next day. He can see that Ralph is coming in tomorrow afternoon for heartburn and chest pain.

Dr. Smith wonders when he last saw Ralph in the clinic. He opens Ralph's medical record in the ambulatory clinical system to look at Ralph's last clinic note. Dr. Smith can also see **notes and multidisciplinary documentation from other UAB clinics and the hospital.** He reviewed the note from Gastroenterology detailing Ralph's last colonoscopy, as well as **scanned notes** from Ralph's previous internist who was not a part of the UAB system. After Dr. Smith concludes his review, he calls it a day and heads home. Ralph arrives the next day, right on time for his appointment. He identifies himself with a

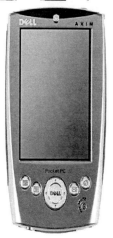

thumbprint scan at the front desk. At this time Ralph receives his **schedule of diagnostic procedures.** After Ralph completes his lab work, he returns to Dr. Smith's office and is quickly called back by Dr. Smith's nurse, Julie.

Julie has a **hand-held device** with her that allows her to access Ralph's record from anywhere in the clinic. She opens his record, where she can see Ralph's **allergies that were documented at his last visit.** She verifies with Ralph that he has "no known allergies." As she weighs and measures Ralph, the values are automatically collected by the system. The **system performs calculations** such as BSA and BMI that can be displayed later for Dr. Smith and other departments such as pharmacy.

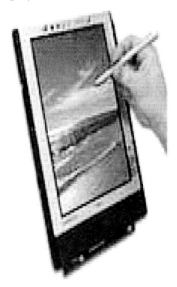

Julie escorts Ralph to the exam room and accesses the clinical system on the **wireless tablet PC.** The system displays Ralph's chief complaint, so Julie can quickly and easily pull up a corresponding **exam template** for Dr. Smith. Dr. Smith enters the room and completes the History of Present Illness and Review of Systems in the template quickly, using options such as **check boxes, pick-lists, and "shortcuts"** that replace abbreviations with larger pieces of text. Even though there are documentation templates available for multiple conditions/specialties, Dr. Smith still utilizes **voice recognition dictation** from time to time, especially for new patient visits.

Dr. Smith proceeds to examine Ralph thoroughly. When Dr. Smith is finished he **enters orders** for Ralph. Dr. Smith is pretty sure Ralph has reflux disease, but does not want to dismiss his chest pain. He reviews **evidence-based guidelines** for current research information, and then orders a **standard cardiac workup,** which includes multiple tests such as an EKG, a CBC, and cardiac enzymes to rule out anything more serious. After he enters the order, he is **prompted for a diagnosis for each.** Not only is the diagnosis associated with the order for medical necessity, but Ralph's **problems list is simultaneously updated for this visit!**

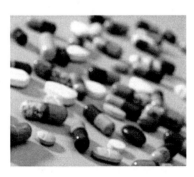

Additionally, as Dr. Smith enters radiology/lab orders, **ABN checking is performed.** The system **alerts** Dr. Smith that Medicare will not cover the tests ordered for "gastric reflux." At this point the system allows Dr. Smith the option to access the local medical review policy (LMRP). Dr. Smith discusses this with Ralph and Ralph agrees that the testing is needed. Dr. Smith also **orders a referral** to Dr. Jones at the cardiology clinic and finishes his orders by **prescribing** Nexium for Ralph.

Dr. Smith is able to select Nexium from his **"favorites" medication list** and he is quickly **alerted that Ralph has no allergies to it.** However, he is also **alerted that Nexium is not in Medicare's preferred formulary.** Dr. Smith **searches the electronic drug information** and changes the order to Prilosec, which is automatically updated to Ralph's current medications list. Ralph mentions he is low on Zyrtec. Dr. Smith picks Zyrtec from Ralph's current medications list, where he's able to **see the complete prescribing history, including strength, dose, number of refills, and so forth.** With a couple of screen taps, Dr. Smith is able to **refill** Ralph's Zyrtec.

Dr. Smith cannot complete all of his documentation at this time, so he places Ralph's visit note in a "suspended" status to be completed at the end of the day. However, he quickly makes a **handwritten note on the tablet PC.** The handwritten note is **converted to an electronic entry immediately.**

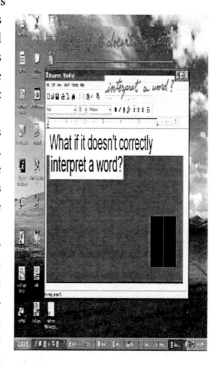

Before Dr. Smith leaves the room, he glances at the **health maintenance reminders** for Ralph. He lets Ralph know that he is due for a prostate screening which will be scheduled for him as he checks out, and because it is flu season, he recommends a flu shot as well.

Julie enters the room one last time to administer the flu shot. She provides Ralph with a **patient education form on flu vaccines, which she was able to print from the clinical system.** She administers the vaccine and uses a standard immunization EMAR or a clinic **documentation template** to quickly document lot number, site, expiration date, and patient response.

Julie escorts Ralph to the checkout area, where the checkout clerk advises him of his financial responsibility for his lab/radiology tests. Ralph signs the ABN form using **the electronic signature stylus** and the appointments are then scheduled for lab and radiology, as well as the appointment with Dr. Jones. The checkout clerk also informs Ralph that his prescriptions were **sent electronically to the retail pharmacy of his choice.** This information was obtained when Ralph updated his health record.

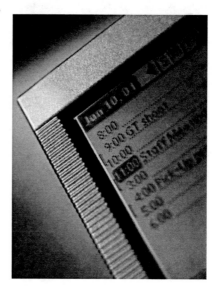

The day after Ralph's visit, Dr. Smith logs onto the clinical system to complete Ralph's clinic visit note. Once he has completed the note, Dr. Smith can verify that his note satisfies the Level of Service (LOS) using **Evaluation and Management criteria in the system.**

After Dr. Smith signs the note, the encounter information (diagnosis, LOS, CPT codes) is **sent electronically to the billing system** automatically.

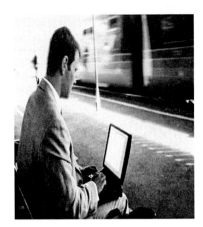

As a courtesy, Dr. Smith sends Ralph's clinic note to Dr. Jones's inbox in the clinical system. Dr. Jones, the cardiologist, **accesses the ambulatory clinical system from anywhere** and sees the note. He quickly accesses Ralph's record to enter. Dr. Jones or a member of his team then calls Ralph to let him know he needs to go to the hospital for further testing and evaluation.

.....to be continued (in the acute care optimal story)

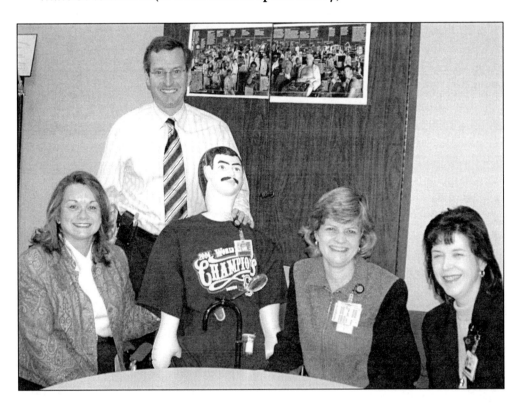

UAB Core Clinical Project Team Members:
Rhonda Callander, CIO Mike Waldrum, "Ralph," Gretchen Kennamer and Melanie Turner.

APPENDIX 2-2
SAMPLE IT PROJECT COMMUNICATION PLAN

Communication Management Plan
for the Core Clinicals System
(PIN Replacement Project)

(Date)

Summary of Contents

1. Project Background
2. Communication Management Plan
   A. Resources
      Project Management Team
      Communications Team
      Stakeholders
   B. Methods of Communicating
   C. Reporting
   D. Communication Paths
   E. Project Library
   F. Communication Basics
3. Communication Matrix

Project Background

The University of Alabama Birmingham Health System (UABHS) is Alabama's principal tertiary healthcare provider, serving local, regional, national, and international patients with state-of-the-science treatment modalities. Each component of UABHS supports its threefold mission of patient care, teaching, and research.

UABHS continues its initiative to improve patient care and satisfaction across the health system. One area of focus includes the need to replace the Patient Information Network (PIN) with a comprehensive system that offers advanced and integrated functionality.

The scope of this project plan will focus on:
- Capturing and objectively presenting UAB's desired Future State and specific business objectives
- Planning for organizational change, including developing and implementing an organizational communication plan.

This project will include all hospital areas that are touched by the current Patient Information Network system, as well as The Kirklin Clinic (TKC) and outlying clinics. This will include, but is not limited to, functionality for acute care, ambulatory, pharmacy, medication management, clinical documentation, orders and results, and rules and alerts.

The scope of the "Core Clinical System" for the purpose of this project includes:
- Orders Management
- Decision Support

- Results Reporting
- Clinical Documentation
- Medication Management
- Pharmacy
- Health Information Management

The significance of the Core Clinical System as the foundation for quality care delivery cannot be overemphasized. The functionality of the system has a direct impact on patient safety, patient satisfaction, quality care delivery, medical education, and clinical research.

PIN has been in successful operation serving the enterprise needs for over 10 years, but it is built on technology that limits its continued enhancement. It also lacks specific key functionality that is currently needed in the complex UABHS healthcare environment. UABHS desires to replace this current system with a state of the art system that addresses patient care alerts, provider orders management, clinical documentation, pharmacy requirements, and complete medication administration management, including electronic medication administration records (EMAR).

Communication Management Plan

The large scale embedded user base of the PIN system drives the need for a coherent communication plan that will provide the key stakeholders with the appropriate level of project information, as well as reach the user population as a whole.

Communication provides the necessary links and cohesion between team members, stakeholders, users, and management. The communication plan will be used as a guide for creating and distributing the project information. A good communication plan defines what information will be developed, who will develop the information, how and when the information will be produced, and to whom the information will be distributed. The purpose of the communication plan is to:

- Set and manage expectations
- Develop awareness
- Obtain cooperation
- Establish ownership
- Provide status
- Provide a forum for feedback
- Ensure consistent interpretation of information

Resources: Project Management Team

Rhonda Callander	Project Manager
Melanie Turner	Acute Care
Gretchen Kennamer	Ambulatory

Resources: Communication Team

Lynn Graves	PMT/Communication Lead
Gretchen Kennamer	PMT/ HSIS PIN expert
Melanie Turner	PMT/ HSIS PIN expert
Rhonda Callander	PMT
	Medical Doctors
Patrice Jones	Nurses
	Ancillary Departments
	Pharmacy
	Training / Staff Development
	Media Specialists
	Research
	Academics (School of Medicine)
	TKC

Resources: Stakeholders

Dr. Mike Waldrum	Chief Information Officer, Project Champion
Dr. Nancy Dunlap	Chief of Staff TKC, Project Champion
Cynthia Barginere	Chief Nursing Officer, Project Champion
Joan Hicks	HSIS Director
Don Fast	HSIS Director
Herb Smaltz	Chief Technology Officer
	Executives
	AEDs
	Department Directors
	HSIS
	Department Chairs
	MD Advisory Group
	Residents
	Nursing
	Unit Secretaries
	Pharmacy
	Ancillaries
	Staff Development
	NIST
	Physicians
	Board members
	Research
	Academics

Methods of Communicating

A communication matrix detailing the information recipients and the communication methods (memos, verbal, e-mail, meetings, publications, etc.) has been developed and is located at the end of this Appendix. The communication matrix contains the individuals or groups involved with the project, the types of information required, and the dates accomplished. The purpose of the communication matrix is to ensure the creation of the proper information and the accurate and timely distribution of created information to the appropriate parties.

Another important aspect of communication is the interaction among the project team members, owner(s), and other project stakeholders. On all major projects, communication is needed among all project stakeholders. The use of advisory teams, user groups, and newsletters can also help to ensure the client community's expectations are developed and realized. The project manager must understand the importance of communication to the success of the project and create an environment in which communication is encouraged and accomplished. Both external and internal communication must be included in the communication plan.

Reporting

Project Management Team (PMT) meetings are held weekly to discuss progress, existing or evolving issues that may have been encountered, and the updating of previously assigned action items. These items are documented in the weekly status report. The Communication Team Lead will attend the PMT meetings and provide a progress report for inclusion in the weekly status report.

Communication Paths

A project team environment presents communication challenges. It is particularly important that communication paths be established among the team, the project stakeholders and the clinicians. It is recognized that the communication tasks become more difficult with a larger project team membership. Project communications will be oral, written, and nonverbal.

Presentations are formally made to executive stakeholders utilizing Microsoft PowerPoint presentations. Design sessions are used to elicit information from a targeted group of participants. Review sessions will be used to present the proposed vision and are open to the vast majority of the user population. An intranet Web page has been created to further spread the word about the project. Articles have been written and approved for publishing in various UAB newsletters and magazines.

Project Library

Project documentation serves as the project's knowledge base and is called the project library. The library includes documents, work products, support tools, standards and deliverables. The library provides an account of project activities, information, decisions, and status. All knowledge of the project will be captured in the library where any authorized individual, (internal or external [Read Only] to the project), can go to retrieve project information and products. The library can be located on the shared drive using the following path: \\hossvc01\vol2\DPTS\HIS\Projects\PIN Replacement.

Communication Basics

- Communication between team members will be on a continuous basis.
- Educate all constituencies on what the project is and is not.
- Be honest about how the project is going to progress and about possible outcomes; do not make unrealistic promises (e.g., no one's job will change).
- Teammates will communicate face-to-face, as well as via e-mail, pager and telephone.
- Weekly status meetings will be held to discuss project progress, deliverables, issues, risks, action items and other items as they become necessary.
- Standardized templates will be used for document creation and posted into the repository.
- Establish a regular schedule for communicating and stick to it; do not start a regular mechanism and then get too busy to continue it.
- Additional meetings will be held on an as-needed basis.
- All meeting minutes and supporting documentation will be kept in the repository.
- All communication with the stakeholders or contract vendors will be documented and stored in the repository.

Communication Matrix

The communication matrix provides a vehicle for documenting the necessary information for timely and useful communication within the impacted areas. The columns are populated with the following information:

- Identifies stakeholders as any constituency impacted.
- Defines goals and objectives for communication to each stakeholder group.
- Identifies the medium to be used based on stakeholder needs (publications, presentation at standing meetings, posters, e-mailings, and Web sites [Horizon, SCR]).
- Defines the specific content information, specific to each group or area.
- Defines the timeframe in which to communicate.
- Specifies any issues or details about the particular communication item; identifies the responsible person for each communication milestone.

These tasks will be tracked in the project plan, which will monitor the progress and identify any gaps.

Vision Phase

	PIN Replacement Communication Plan				
Stakeholder	Objective	Plan/Medium	Content	Timing	Responsible Person & Activity
Leadership Executive Management	Inform on cost/benefits, service, quality, milestone completion	• Meeting verbal update • Slides	• Brief status update • Outcomes	• Operations Oversight Team -at completion of vision	**Mike Waldrum** • ITAG 9/20 • Mgmt Forum (email) 9/22 • OOT
Leadership— Project Steering Team	To keep informed, resolve issues, make decisions as needed	• Schedule time PRN at weekly AED meeting • Decision Day 1 • Decision Day 2	• Inform on methodology • Update of progress • Prepare for Decision Days/ other milestones • Include educational information during retreat— Marion Ball, speaker on 'Revolution in Healthcare Transformation' • Outcomes	• Prior to milestones • PRN	**PMT** • Decision Day 1 with "retreat" 10/13, 1–5pm • Decision Day 2
Leadership — Office of the CIO	To keep informed, resolve issues, make decisions as needed	• Weekly status report	• Accomplishments • Pending activities • Issues/risks	• Weekly	**Rhonda Callander**

PIN Replacement Communication Plan

Stakeholder	Objective	Plan/Medium	Content	Timing	Responsible Person & Activity
Nursing	Increase awareness, engage in Design Sessions, keep informed	• NIST Team • Nurse Educator Group • Sr. Nursing Leadership Council • Communications book • Unit meetings • *Monday Mailing* • *Computer Tutor* • *Nursing Matters* • Intranet Web site • eHealth	• Initial introduction to method and project • Updates as appropriate • Design Session participation • Educational information • Final outcome	• Ongoing during project • SNLC – 2nd & 4th Tues	**Melanie Turner/ Gretchen Kennamer** • Articles delivered to SME's 9/7 • Sr. Nursing Leadership 9/21 • Nurse Mgrs 9/28 • NIST (email) 9/? • *Monday Mailing 9/24* 9/23
Medical Staff	Increase awareness, engage in Design Sessions, keep informed	• *UAB Synopsis* • Medical Executive Committee • Clinical Council Meeting • Clinic chairs	• Initial introduction to method and project • Updates as appropriate • Design Session participation • Educational information • Final outcome	• Monthly • Periodic	• **PMT** – *UAB Synopsis* 10/11 • **Mike Waldrum** - Clinical Council 9/7 • **Nancy Dunlap** - Clinic Chairs 9/14
All employees (UAB)	Increase awareness, keep informed	• *Grapevine (Ambulatory)*	• Initial introduction to method and project • Updates as appropriate • Final outcome		**Gretchen Kennamer**
All employees (TKC)	Increase awareness, keep informed	• *Monday Mailing (Hospital)*	• Initial introduction to method and project • Updates as appropriate • Final outcome		**Melanie Turner** 9/24

PIN Replacement Communication Plan

Stakeholder	Objective	Plan/Medium	Content	Timing	Responsible Person & Activity
Managers	Increase awareness, keep informed	• Senior Managers Meeting - clinic medical directors and clinic managers • Management Forum— dept directors and nursing managers	• Initial introduction to method and project • Updates as appropriate • Final outcome	• Sr. Mgrs Mtg - 1st and 3rd Friday of each month; 10:30-11:30 5th floor conference room in TKC • Mgmt Forum	**Melanie Turner/ Gretchen Kennamer**
Pharmacy	Increase awareness, keep informed	• Dept meetings	• Initial introduction to method and project • Updates as appropriate • Final outcome		
Residents	Increase awareness, keep informed	House Staff Council Surgery Grand Rounds	• Initial introduction to method and project • Updates as appropriate • Final outcome		**Melanie Turner/ Gretchen Kennamer**
All	Increase awareness, keep informed	• https://scr.hs.uab.edu/ vision • Horizon	• Session schedule • Optimal stories • Feedback form • Progress updates	9/23 Go-live Monthly progress updates	**Rhonda Callander**

Acknowledgments

Special thanks to the UAB Health System Core Clinical Replacement Project team members Rhonda Callandar (UAB), Melanie Turner (UAB), Gretchen Kennamer (UAB), Heidi Wurtz (Healthlink Incorporated) and Alan Bowen (Healthlink Incorporated) for providing a sample project vision statement and communication plan.

References

1. Feeny D, Edwards B, Simpson K: Understanding the CEO/CIO Relationship. *MIS Quarterly.* Dec. 1992; 435–447.
2. Brier T: So You Want to Be a CIO. *3X-400 Systems Management.* 1994; 22(8): 66–69.
3. Palmlund D: In Search of the Ideal CIO. *Financial Executive.* 1997; 13(3): 37–39.
4. CIO Position Description. CIO Magazine.1997; available at www.cio.com/CIO/re_posit.htm, CIO Communications, Inc.
5. Wang C: Technovision: *The Executive's Guide to Understanding and Managing Information Technology.* New York, NY: McGraw-Hill; 1994.
6. Hayden F: A Mars/Pluto Relationship. *Optimize Magazine.* Jan. 2002; Issue 22; available at http://www.optimizemag.com.
7. King J: Chasm Closer: The CIO/CEO Gap Still Dogs IS. *Computerworld.* 1995; 29(21): 84–85.
8. Klug L: Hatred: An Update (CIO-CEO Relationships). *Forbes.* 1996; 158(8): 100–104.
9. Wang C: *Technovision II : Every Executive's Guide to Understanding and Mastering Technology and the Internet.* New York, NY: McGraw-Hill; 1997.
10. Wilder C: CIOs Not Up to Snuff as Active Business Leaders. *Computerworld.* 1992; 26(11): 6.
11. Smaltz D: Elevating CIO Roles: Organizational Barriers and Organizational Enablers. *Journal of Healthcare Information Management.* Spring 2000; 14(1): 81–91.
12. Kaplan RS, Norton DP: *The Balanced Scorecard,* Boston, MA: Harvard Business School Press; 1996.

CHAPTER 3

Crystal Balls: The Elusive Art of Business and IT Strategic Alignment

Rulon F. Stacey, PhD, and Richard I. Skinner, MS, MHA, FCHIME

One of the trustees called Sam Weatherspoon to discuss a strategic planning meeting that had occurred the week before. The meeting had focused on a range of issues confronting Ingalls: lowering the costs of operations, addressing nursing shortage and morale issues, and developing an outpatient strategy in the southern suburbs.

The trustee, the CEO of a local bank, had commented on his organization's strategy development process. He noted how important IT was to their ability to execute their strategy. He asked Sam about the IT implications of the Ingalls strategy. Sam frowned and answered that he didn't know. IT was certainly busy and was spending a lot of money, but it wasn't clear to him that those efforts were advancing the strategy.

By now, everyone knows about strategic alignment between an organization's business strategy and IT. It's lesson number one in any CIO's training, always a topic of conversation in any gathering of CIOs, and the subject of numerous articles. Figure 3-1 is an example of how Providence Health System's Regional Information Services Group views the alignment of business strategy and IT.

But do organizations really achieve that alignment, or even understand what it is? In many, if not most cases, the answer is "no." And that negative answer is one of the major reasons why IT has yet to achieve the kind of success in supporting the healthcare industry that it has in virtually every other industry.

THE CEO PERSPECTIVE

While it is true that synergy of purpose may align all parties toward the same goal, the CEO's vision of an organization is often different than that of the CIO and others in the IT group. To the CEO, the question is not always a matter of aligning the parties toward the same goal; more often the question is, "How does one align the incentives of different parties toward achieving the same goal?"

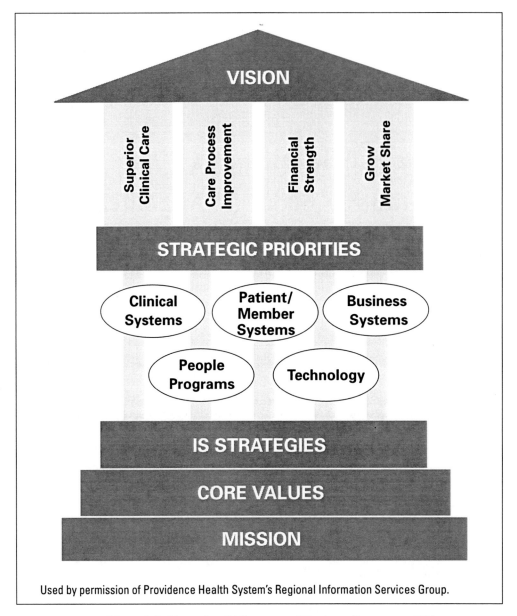

Figure 3-1. Example of Alignment of Business Strategy and IT

In asking this question, the CEO of a hospital or a health system is asking a question that is no different than has to be asked in all other departments of the organization. This same question is asked a hundred times a day throughout the organization in determining how to coordinate a new service line with the marketing department, or how to upgrade the surgical wing without offending the family physician, or anyone of the other hundred decisions that must be made.

In creating synergy between departments, the challenges faced by the IT department are no different than the challenges of any other department; specifically, the challenges which impact the creation of new IT programs are seldom any different than those in other areas of the organization. And, because the challenges are the same, the solutions are also the same, and the solution centers on the leadership ability of the IT executive, or the ability of the IT leader to understand the entire organization and implement change as a part of the whole, and resist the temptation to view IT as independent of other parts of the organization.

It is no longer enough for a CIO to know only about information technology. In today's environment, a CIO must know much more, including how to be an accomplished leader not only for IT but also for the entire organization. IT is much more than simply implementing certain projects; it is creating a strategy that meets the needs of the organization and then providing the leadership necessary to carry this forward within the framework of the overall organization.

STRATEGIC ALIGNMENT DEFINED

What exactly is strategic alignment? We can start with what it is not. Strategic alignment is not IT taking technology orders from its customers. Certainly the customers would like their orders fulfilled, but simply doing so makes IT, by definition, a tactic, not a discipline with strategic value. On the other hand, IT is not a strategy by itself, at least not a successful one in healthcare. While it has transformed other industries and been the foundation for success of numerous companies, this has not been the case in healthcare. It could happen, but most healthcare organizations probably do not want to risk being first.

Real strategic alignment between healthcare strategy and IT is just that, an alignment of the strengths of each, employed to achieve business purposes. It begins with synergy of purpose, that is: "what are we trying to achieve"; involves mutual development of goals and plans to achieve them ("let's work together"); and always involves shared accountability ("we're in this together"). If these elements are present, there is a much greater likelihood that business projects will have appropriate IT support and that IT projects will appropriately support business goals.

In the following sections, we will examine each of these elements from both the CEO and CIO perspective. We will also use some examples to demonstrate the value of these elements in achieving strategic alignment.

SYNERGY OF PURPOSE

Synergy of purpose is crucial to teamwork, and the success of IT support to healthcare relies on teamwork. Healthcare is a large collection of different disciplines, people, and priorities, and most healthcare strategies and IT initiatives must coordinate all of them to be successful. A successful information system implementation as viewed by the IT department is quite different than that viewed by the lab, nursing or some other part of the organization, and yet both have to be successful in order to produce business value.

This section will present some examples of IT/business initiatives to demonstrate the effect of synergy of purpose. The first is a project to implement (a) a simplified, more customer friendly registration process, or (b) a new computer system called an enterprise master patient index, which will match patients seen in the outpatient/ physician office setting with those seen in an inpatient/hospital setting.

In this example, a large, multi-hospital, multi-practice integrated delivery system discovered that the registration processes in its owned practices, hospital-based outpatient services, and inpatient services were all quite different and forced patients and staff to collect information multiple times. This resulted in redundant work and customer inconvenience. The proposed solution was to implement a new information system, called an enterprise master patient index, so that at the point of registration, information previously given to the health system in another setting could be used to register the patient in a different setting.

As it was discovered, this was an information system solution to a business process problem. The health system desired a simpler registration process, which would make use of information previously collected in other settings and information systems. However, the IT goal was the implementation of a master patient index system, which in and of itself would not achieve the business goal. The result was the mostly successful implementation of a master patient index system that failed to produce a simplified multi-setting registration process. Despite best intentions on both sides, and a very high organizational priority, the initiative did not meet its objectives, simply because the objectives were never defined in the same way for all parties.

A second example is the implementation of a physician office-based electronic medical record system. In this case, the project goal was to implement an electronic medical record system that would supply the data to enable the medical group to better manage its population of patients. It was quite clear from the onset that improved population health management in the physician office setting was the long-term goal of the project. While short-term productivity increases and other cost savings were desirable, the long-term goal was paramount and the project would not be successful until that goal was achieved.

This was good news for the IT department in that initial implementation problems were tolerated and its customer was focused on the strategic value of the system, not on short-term results. However, it was also bad news in that simply making the new system work technically was not sufficient to achieve the project's goals. The IT department not only had to implement the system but ensure it was collecting the right information, and that the same or subsequent systems would be able to use the data to accurately support population health management objectives.

For the medical group, the strategic goal of population health management helped them to weather the initial implementation issues, to maintain their commitment to the project, and ultimately to ensure that both their processes and their information systems were changed in ways that would allow them to reach that goal. While it took five years to implement the system and use its data to better manage the medical group's patient populations, having both the IT department and the medical group focused on the same goal enabled them to work as a team during the project, and to make the decisions and compromises that finally resulted in a successful health system strategic initiative.

Synergy of purpose, or sharing the same goal, gets all parties pointed in the same direction at the beginning of a strategic initiative or project, but it does not ensure that they will continue to work in concert toward the same goal. In order to have continuous alignment, all parties must be involved in the day-to-day administration and decision-making functions of the project.

Projects—IT or others—are all subject to entropy. That is, left alone, they will tend toward chaos. So, ensuring that mechanisms are in place to continually make certain that all parties are involved in setting goals, working toward those goals, and monitoring and reporting progress along the way, is critical to maintaining alignment during the course of any strategic initiative. The following example explores a situation where continuous coordination between the parties involved in an IT-based strategic initiative resulted in success.

In this example, after an initial period of poor communication between the IT department and the surgery department, the two organizations decided they would have to work much more closely together to design and implement IT systems to support a large new operating room (OR) construction project. The surgery department had committed to a new process model for the new ORs that would result in increased productivity but which was heavily dependent on the use of new information technology such as device and patient locating systems, electronic scheduling boards, and others.

Both departments realized that in order to be successful, both the new technology and new processes would have to be designed to support each other. To that end, an integrated project team was formed and that team developed the project plan for all aspects of the project. As both the technology and business processes were new to the project team, the project plan changed greatly during the course of the project, but because those changes and decisions were made through close coordination within the team, the project goals were maintained and the team remained focused on achieving them.

At the conclusion of the project, not only had the ORs been built, the information systems installed, and the business processes redesigned, but all of them worked well together and resulted in the project achieving its goals. This outcome could not have happened if there had been separate IT and surgery project teams, or if within the project team, the IT staff simply installed whatever technology surgery wanted, or if surgery had no say in the technology choices made by IT. It was the close, day-to-day coordination within the team that kept goals shared and work complimentary as the project evolved.

However, even with synergy of purpose and mutual development of goals and plans, IT and business alignment is impossible to achieve without shared accountability. Shared accountability means all parties involved in a strategic initiative or project are responsible not just for their own portion of the project, but for the overall success of the project.

While the concept of shared accountability in healthcare is widely discussed and accepted, in practice it is very difficult to get people and organizations to share accountability for results when they do not each control all the resources. The same thing is true in business initiatives that use IT. All too often it is the IT department's role simply to install the system and the business department's role to just use the new system. Even if both parties achieve their goals individually, the goal of the project to produce business value for the organization may not be met. It is only when neither partly can be successful without the other party also being successful, and that both parties are held accountable to a shared goal, that true shared accountability is present. And that shared accountability is the major predictor for IT projects producing real business value.

EXAMPLES OF THE VALUE OF SHARED ACCOUNTABILITY

The following two examples will illustrate the value of shared accountability in achieving strategy alignment. The first describes an initiative to produce improved documentation and nursing productivity through the use of a clinical documentation system, and the second describes a project to reduce administrative costs in finance, human resources and materials management through the implementation of an integrated Enterprise Resource Planning System (ERP).

Example-Clinical Documentation System

In the first example, as part of the formation of an integrated delivery system, a hospital was to change its complete set of information systems in order to become "standard" with the rest of the health system. In human resources, finance, patient accounting and other support services, the change in information systems was a necessary first step toward consolidation of those services for the health system, with clear benefits.

However, one of the systems to be implemented, as the hospital converted, was a nursing documentation system, which previously had not existed at that hospital. It was added to the family of systems to be implemented because the other hospitals in the system used it and it seemed to make sense to the executive team and to the IT department to standardize on this system as part of the overall project. The nursing department was convinced to support this strategy and was interested in using IT in its operations. However, from the beginning of the project, the hospital's nursing leadership was only accountable for supporting the implementation of the documentation system, not for its use or producing value from it.

While the nursing department contributed staff to the project and, at considerable expense, trained over 1,000 nurses to use the system, its goal was simply participation, not achieving benefits. The documentation system implementation encountered numerous technical issues that caused the nursing department to question the value of the system, and ultimately to decide that whatever value the system might have, it did not outweigh the implementation headaches they were experiencing. Ultimately the system was de-installed and it would be an additional eight years before it was reintroduced into that hospital.

While the technical issues were real, disruptive, and took time to resolve, the nursing department measured their impact against the benefit of simply participating in the project. This made a decision to abandon the system a relatively easy one. The IT department was accountable for installing the system, not nursing, and no one was accountable for achieving any business benefit from the system. Had both departments been made jointly accountable for achieving demonstrated value from the new system, the outcome might have been different.

Example-Enterprise Resource Planning System

In the second example, a healthcare system made the decision to implement a replacement information system for its aging financial, human resources, and procurement systems. Furthermore, because multiple facilities and regions within the organization had the same issues with aging systems, the decision was made to implement the same new information system, with "standard" data and structures (general ledger, vendor master, job codes, and so on) in all the regions and facilities. This joint implementation of a new information system was to be the first time that the health system had attempted a cross-regional project of any type.

While the goal for the project initially was simply to replace the existing system with one standard new system, the health system recognized that the impact of so doing would be substantial and would have to be managed from a business perspective, not just an IT systems implementation perspective. To ensure all parties were involved and accountable, the executives leading the finance and human resource departments, as well as the CIOs, were made jointly accountable for the success of the project. Because of this joint accountability (and explicit objectives linked to compensation), the executives had the incentive to form an active project steering council to provide oversight and support to the project and to encourage their teams to work through the many issues encountered during the project. The system was successfully implemented, but during the process, many contentious issues surfaced that only a sense of shared accountability could, and did, solve. That shared accountability was the "glue" that held the project and the team together.

THE CEO PERSPECTIVE

In leading the IT process, an effective IT senior executive should remember five things:
1. Hospitals are the most complex organizations in existence today;
2. Existing systems are usually sufficient;
3. The user is always right;
4. The user is never right; and
5. Good IT executives develop an understanding of numbers 3 and 4.

Hospitals Are the Most Complex Organizations in Existence Today

In the February 2002 issue of the *Harvard Business Review*, Peter Drucker, arguably the greatest organizational mind of our time, said that hospitals are the most complex organizations ever devised. That is no small statement. Having studied all different types of organizations, Drucker should know. One challenge of an IT executive is to make everyone in the IT department, especially those in leadership roles, understand this fact.

The fact that someone may know IT does not mean that they know healthcare IT. The nuances of working in a hospital setting are different than anything else an IT person will work through. The politics are different, the personalities more volatile, the differences between departments more pronounced. Everything is harder, and without that understanding and willingness to work through these more difficult circumstances, an IT person will never be successful in healthcare. No CIO should assume for a minute that you can hire someone and that person will be successful just because they know IT. They have to be able to demonstrate the patience necessary to be successful in healthcare and the aptitude to learn the differences inherent in healthcare.

Existing Systems Are Usually Sufficient

Clinical and IT people alike seem to share the need to bring in new systems just for the sake of having new systems. There are many examples (many of them personal) of hospitals and health systems implementing new IT projects that require hundreds of hours of training for the staff to fully understand the new system. But if the staff had spent hundreds of hours training on the old system, it would have worked just fine, without the cost of implementing a new system. The effective leadership discussed below will go a long way toward correcting this problem. We do not have the luxury in healthcare to spend the extra money or time to create a solution that could be achieved much more easily and less expensively by simply putting in the time and effort to understand the current system.

The User Is Always Right

This is one of the fundamental challenges for IT leadership. And, when an understanding of this principle is combined with the information immediately following, it will enable the IT leader to better understand the complexity of the organization as well as the need for leadership skills. In order to be successful, an IT function must meet the needs of the customer it is trying to serve. In this case, the customer is the end user of the product— the nurse, patient registrar, physician, or whomever may be in need of the system or product. Successful IT executives will understand this concept and treat the end user as a customer, every bit as much as patients are treated as customers, physicians are treated as customers, or as retail shoppers are treated as customers by Wal-Mart.

The User Is Never Right

Herein lies the challenge. The user is the customer and needs to be treated as such. The customer is always right. The problem is that the customer rarely, if ever, fully understands what IT products they need to be successful. All they know is that they want to have the greatest ease possible when working with their patients or the medical record or the registration system. They want efficiency and comfort. While they think they know what it will take to achieve these things, they are usually far too naïve on the technical details to fully understand their own needs. They may have looked at a brochure at a professional meeting or talked to a colleague or friend and think they know what they want and need. However, they usually know little or nothing of the complexity of the greater needs of the organization or what will or will not work with the overall IT components in the organization.

Therefore, the task of the talented IT executive is to know how to meet the needs of people who don't know what they need, and to make those people believe that they thought of the solution in the first place. If this challenge sounds daunting, it is. Nevertheless, the CEO faces this dilemma every day when trying to make one facility understand the need to financially support another, or when the surgery department gets a new intensive care unit when the medical unit cannot. This is the challenge of leadership, and for IT, it will fall squarely on the shoulders of the IT executive to ensure that this challenge is met. Only a good IT executive will be able to achieve this.

Good IT Executives Understand This Seeming Contradiction

An understanding of this seeming contradiction does not come from a background in IT alone. While an IT background is most beneficial, the successful IT executive in this decade must have leadership skills first and foremost. In fact, the best IT executives will have the following characteristics:

Extensive Leadership Training. The best CIOs will have much more than an IT background. They will have formal education in leadership skills as well as an extensive background in IT. An MBA or MHA or equivalent will separate the successful IT executives from the rest. Active participation in the American College of Healthcare Executives will help the IT executive stay on course with the leadership skills that are necessary for success.

Extensive IT Background and Training. The leadership skills described above are exceptionally important. Those are the skills that will enable IT executives to transfer their knowledge to the organization in a collaborative and facilitative manner, as opposed to forcing the decision on a group of people who have yet to buy into the process. However, without the specific background in IT to know what the organization needs and how the industry is capable of helping the organization, the IT executive is not as valuable as otherwise might be. It is critical for the executive to be well versed in the technical side of the job. This is why the IT executive of the next decade will be in such demand. Those who are able to master all of these various skill sets will be in critical demand, but in very short supply.

Organizational Behavior Skills. In the end, the product of the two characteristics described above will be demonstrated by the organizational behavior (OB) skills of the IT executive. The IT executive must know how to select the right people and how to get them to integrate into an already complex organization. For example, in implementing a strategy into an emergency department (ED), the successful IT executive will understand that the physicians (who think themselves superior to the nurses) and the nurses (who think themselves superior to the paramedics) and the paramedics (who think themselves superior to the EMTs) and the EMTs (who think themselves superior to the aides) and the aides all must work toward one common goal.

The successful executive must be able to lead the ED toward the greater good not only of that department but also the entire organization. It is a difficult task to be certain. But the days of an IT executive just being able to know IT and what systems work well are gone. Having a good technical background is simply not enough. One must have a good technical background, but must also have the leadership and interpersonal skills and training to be an effective leader for IT and for the entire organization.

So, these are the basics for creating an exceptional IT executive; one who can help an organization achieve goals that it never before thought possible. But how will this work practically in most healthcare organizations? Recall the example of the formation of an integrated delivery system where one hospital was to be made "standard" with the rest of the organization. In that example it was suggested that if nursing or other departments were held accountable for the installation of the system, then the process would have been more successful.

Using the leadership theories listed above, this scenario can be taken one step further. If the end users are considered customers, then the analogy of holding the nurses and other departments accountable does not work so well. While the goal is admirable, the process suggested in the example is much like Wal-Mart threatening to punish its customers if a new product they (Wal-Mart) introduce is not successful. Such a process would be unthinkable in retail business, yet we can easily fall into that trap by not understanding the critical customer relationship that exists in a healthcare organization.

In Wal-Mart or any other retail company, before a new service is introduced, the company does extensive research to know what exactly it is that the customers want and what the customers are willing to buy. With that information, and using the more detailed information about what products are and are not available (information that the customer does not even know exists), the company creates a new product or service and then spends a great deal of time getting the customer to understand and buy the new product. There is no hint of the company suggesting that the customer be held accountable for the success or failure of the new product or service.

This is true in healthcare organizations as well. If the IT executive believes that there is a better IT system or, in this case, a better way to standardize the integrated delivery system, then it is the job of the IT executive to ensure that the customers (e.g., nurses and doctors) understand the system and that they themselves are "sold" on what it will do. The IT executive will have to do this by marketing, persuasion, politics, learning and leading. It is far too simplistic to suggest that if an organization holds the end users accountable for the installation, then all will go better. At best, what the organization will have is a system that works marginally well surrounded by grumpy people. That is not a formula for success.

By using the leadership techniques described above, the successful IT executive will spend a great deal of time and use a great deal of leadership talent to help the end users "buy into" the concept of the new system. If they are sold on the system, then the system will sell itself. It is simply not enough to suggest that by holding the users accountable all will go better. While gaining the support of the customers is a much more difficult challenge than simply holding them accountable for a process that they may not support, those IT executives with the leadership skills necessary to do this will quickly separate themselves from others in their industry.

The interesting fact here is that the healthcare industry tried in the 1990s to gain an advantage by holding the customers accountable, and it did not work. During the 1990s hospital executives knew that they needed the support of primary care and other physicians to be successful. So the industry tried to mandate that support by buying physician practices. The unfortunate result was unmotivated, employed physicians who proved to be extremely costly. The correct way to get physician buy-in is by treating them as customers and meeting their needs. Successful hospital executives understand this and do it well. Those healthcare executives who are not able to develop these skills will simply not be as successful or in as high demand as those who do.

The same ability to lead divergent groups toward an organization's common good is what will make IT executives and their projects successful. What the healthcare industry needs now are IT executives who can rally a group of customers to the correct course. The industry needs IT executives who have enough technical background to know what it is an organization needs and the leadership and organizational behavior skills to make it happen without having to hold the customer accountable for an IT plan that cannot be otherwise sold. Anyone can mandate accountability and attempt to manufacture support. But that support is fleeting. The successful IT executive will generate that support from within by leading the organization in the right direction and by inspiring the nurses, doctors, registrars and others that the system the IT executive is proposing is the best possible course of action for them as end users. A group of nurses and doctors who are inspired by true leadership will, in the end, be much more successful in implementing and effectively utilizing a new system than they would be if they were simply held accountable to implement the CIO's direction for the organization.

Process for Achieving Strategic Alignment

This chapter has looked at what strategic alignment means and reviewed examples of how synergy of purpose, mutual development of goals and plans, and shared accountability are all necessary for strategic alignment. Although the process for achieving it may seem simplistic (Figure 3-2), that process is really no different than any other decision process.

The first decision is the "what." That is: what is the organization trying to achieve, or what is its intent? Obtaining broad agreement on the "what" will maintain focus on it during the course of the project. The second decision is the "who." If it is not clear who is involved and who is accountable, then the pitfalls described in the previous examples are almost sure to be encountered. The third decision is the "how." Those in IT particularly like to jump to the "how" first, without first knowing the "what" and the "who." The "how" is where much of the work will be, but unless that work is focused on the "what" and led by the "who," it is unlikely to result in success. The "what," "who," and "how" will lead to the intended results if all are in place, made explicit to all stakeholders, and routinely reviewed during the course of the project.

Expectations from Strategic Alignment

What should be expected from strategic alignment once it is achieved? The first result should be integration of people, process and technology. That integration is almost always required to produce business value. The second result should be documented and shared new knowledge within the organization. That new knowledge is in and of itself a source of business value, even if it is difficult to measure. The third result should be additional business value. That will be evident because it should be measurable in the same way any other business value is measured. Measures such as lowered cost, added revenue, increased customer satisfaction, greater market share, etc. should be the goals, not just adding another information system, or enhancing an existing one. If organizations insist on measurable business value from all of its projects, then by extension this creates incentives to achieve synergy of purpose, mutual development of goals and plans, and shared accountability. These will go a long way toward ensuring that business value is actually achieved.

What do we do?
We deliver information!

Who do we deliver it to?
The Oregon Region!

Where do we deliver it?
*Anywhere the customer
needs the information!*

When do we deliver it?
Every day, around the clock!

Why do we do it?
*To support the business!
To improve patient outcomes!
To achieve cost reduction and
   efficiency!
To deliver quality customer service!*

How do we deliver it?
*Standard applications,
   data, and technology!
Reliable, secure, supported,
   and monitored systems!
On the Web!*

Figure 3-2. Process for Achieving Strategic Alignment

CEO CONCLUSION

This section has discussed the need for IT executives of the next decade to be leaders more than just technical wizards. Following the criteria outlined above, an IT executive must learn to lead much more than simply know how to manage. This conclusion is offered from the perspective of a CEO of a healthcare system. The leadership techniques offered in this section are identical to those needed by a CEO to meet the needs of the entire organization. If the IT executive will understand the leadership techniques needed in managing the entire organization, and the need to treat those end users in the organization as customers, then the entire organization will be better off, and IT projects will always be more successful.

CIO CONCLUSION

The CIO, like other members of the executive team, is accountable for the performance of the organization (or lack thereof). To contribute to that performance, the CIO must be a member of the team, and then must optimize the use of technology to create business value. However, the CIO cannot do that alone and cannot do it simply by fulfilling the needs of all customers. Just as the materials manager has difficulty achieving supply economies if every department and physician get to order what they want, so too does the CIO have trouble creating value by simply providing whatever systems the customers want or have money for. It was the Wal-Mart CIO's customers who created business value by using the information provided from the CIO's IT systems to consolidate its supply chain, stock its shelves differently, and implement new business practices. Wal-Mart's commitment to creating that value was a prerequisite to the company making its IT investments. The CIO must truly be a partner to the other members of the executive team. The CEO must hold the entire team accountable for creating business value from services and investments, whether that value is increased revenue from a new MRI or reduced medication errors from a barcode-reading computer system. If both happen, the organization will have the benefit of synergy between its business and IT strategies.

Sam found the IT alignment discussion to be one of the most important in his career. He now understood that alignment needed a senior leadership discussion that clarified the goals and strategies of the organization and that the IT strategy was intertwined in those discussions. He now realized that the team had to ask, during strategy discussions, how will our IT investments help us to achieve our goals?

Sam realized that the goals for the IT agenda were not something that they should delegate solely to the CIO. Rather, the discussion of IT goals was a discussion that involved all of the leadership.

Sam now knew that the entire leadership team shared the accountability for the results of the IT investments. Accountability was not something that the team could place entirely on the shoulders of the IT organization.

Finally, Sam realized that he needed to spend time with his CIO. He had to help his CIO understand Sam's perspectives on leadership, IT, the challenges faced by the organization, and the power of treating users as customers. Alignment was more than linking IT to the organization's strategies; it also involved the CEO and CIO understanding each other's views of the industry and the organization.

Rulon F. Stacey, PhD, is CEO of Poudre Valley Health System, a five-hospital system based in Fort Collins, CO. In 1999 Dr. Stacey received the Robert S. Hudgens Award from the American College of Healthcare Executives as the "Young Healthcare Executive of the Year." In 1992, Dr. Stacey was named one of 12 executives under age 40 "who have taken considerable strides to improve the cost, access and overall quality of healthcare delivery in the United States" by Modern Healthcare *magazine. Dr. Stacey holds a bachelor of science in economics, a masters degree in health administration from Brigham Young University, and a doctor of philosophy in health policy from the University of Colorado.*

Richard I. Skinner, MS, MHA, FCHIME, is Vice President-IS and CIO for the Providence Health System, a $4 billion organization that operates 18 hospitals and a health plan with over 500,000 members, employs over 400 physicians, and manages numerous home health and long term care businesses across the four western states. Mr. Skinner has over 20 years experience in healthcare information systems, including positions as the CIO for hospitals, a medical research laboratory, and project manager for the development and implementation of the Department of Defense's global medical information system. He was the recipient in 1994 of the Healthcare Information Executives Forum Crystal Award for Excellence. He received the John Gall Award for Healthcare CIO of the Year at the 2002 Annual HIMSS Conference & Exhibition.

References
1. Drucker PF: They're Not Employees, They're People. *Harvard Business Review.* 2002; 80(2): 70–77.

CHAPTER 4

Where's the Beef? Part 1: Getting Value from Your IT Investments*

John P. Glaser, PhD, FCHIME, FHIMSS, and David E. Garets, FHIMSS

A meeting to prepare for the budget retreat had focused on criteria for selecting capital projects. Operating margins were going to be tight again and the amount of available new capital was going to be smaller than Sam would like.

Sam thought that the criteria proposed were reasonable: improving patient safety, increasing revenue, decreasing costs, improving service and enhancing care quality. But he worried about the leadership team's ability to compare proposals that led to different value propositions. How do you compare an investment that improves patient safety with one that reduces costs? This was going to be particularly challenging for the IT project proposals that seemed to have a preponderance of "softer outcome" value propositions.

Sam wasn't pleased by his realization that even the prior years' investments in IT projects, which claimed to have significant cost reduction or revenue enhancement outcomes, had not seemed to have resulted in any significant margin improvement.

Where did the projected gains from their IT investments go?

THE INFORMATION TECHNOLOGY VALUE PROBLEM

The leadership of healthcare organizations is often confronted with the challenge of realizing value from their IT investments. The leadership may make a series of observations.

1. The magnitude of their IT operating and capital budgets is large. IT operating may consume 2% to 3% of the total operating budget and IT capital may claim 15% to 30% of all capital. This consumption can be the difference between a negative operating margin and a positive margin. A 15% to 30% IT capital expenditure invariably means that funding for biomedical equipment (which can mean new revenue) and buildings (which can support the growth of clinical services) is diminished.

---

* Portions of this chapter were reprinted from Wager KA, Lee FW, Glaser JP: *Managing Health Care Information Systems: A Practical Approach for Health Care Executives.* San Francisco, CA: Jossey Bass; 2005. This material is used by permission of John Wiley & Sons, Inc.

2. The projected growth in IT budgets exceeds the growth in other budget categories. Provider organizations may permit overall operating budgets to increase at a rate close to the medical inflation rate. However, expenditures on IT often experience growth rates of an additional 2% to 5%. At some point, an organization will note that the IT budget growth rate may single-handedly lead to insolvency.
3. Regardless of the amount spent, the leadership feels that the demand is insatiable. Worthwhile proposals go unfunded every year. Infrastructure replacement and upgrades seem never ending.
4. It is difficult to evaluate IT budget requests. At times this difficulty is a reflection of a poorly written or fatuous proposal. However, it can be difficult to compare a proposal that is directed to improve service with one directed to improve care quality with one directed to increase revenue with one necessary to achieve some level of regulatory compliance.
5. The leadership may return blank stares when asked "List three instances over the last five years where IT investments have resulted in clear and unarguable returns to the organization." However, the conversation may be difficult to stop when asked "List three major IT investment disappointments that have occurred over the last five years."

Why does this happen? And what can be done to improve the return on the IT investment?

This chapter explores the challenges of IT value. It will cover several areas:
- The nature of IT value
- Why the IT investment fails to deliver returns
- Achieving sustained, high levels of IT-enabled value
- Management practices for increasing the delivery of IT value

THE NATURE OF IT VALUE

IT value, while potentially significant, can be complex and difficult to measure.

IT Value Can Be Tangible and Intangible

IT can be applied to revenue cycle processes leading to tangible reductions in the claims error queue and days in accounts receivables. Computerized provider order entry (CPOE) can lead to measurable improvements in medication error rates. Web-based access to test results can lead to significant gains in result turnaround times.

Cost accounting systems can lead to improved decision making. Electronic mail systems can enhance communication. A system that supports the management of patients with chronic disease can, for example, increase organizational competency in treating this class of patients. These gains are real but intangible: very difficult, if not impossible, to measure.

The Value Can Be Significant

Glaser[1] described the return achieved by replacing the manual approach to determining patient eligibility for coverage with an approach based on electronic data interchange (EDI). One hospital estimated that for an initial investment of $250,000 in eligibility interface development and rollout effort, plus an annual maintenance fee of $72,000, it could achieve ongoing annual savings of approximately $485,000. The EDI investment return was achieved within a year of operation.

Wang[2] analyzed the costs and benefits of the electronic medical record in primary care. This rather sophisticated analysis explored the return over a range of electronic medical record capabilities (from basic to advanced), practice sizes (small to large) and reimbursement structures (from entirely fee for service to extensive risk sharing arrangements). On average the net estimated benefit was $86,000 per provider over five years.

Bates[3] found a 55% reduction in serious medication errors that resulted from the implementation of inpatient CPOE at the Brigham and Women's Hospital. The order entry system highlighted, at the time of ordering, possible drug allergies, drug-drug interactions and drug-lab result problems.

These examples, and many others, demonstrate that IT can be applied to achieve significant gains in organizational performance.

Value Can Be Diverse Across IT Proposals

Consider three proposals that might be in front of the leadership for consideration.

*A **Disaster Notification System**.* This would enable the organization to page critical personnel and inform them that a disaster had taken place (e.g., a train wreck or biotoxin outbreak), the extent of the disaster, and the steps that they need to take to help the organization to respond to the disaster. The system would cost $520,000. The value would be "better preparedness for a disaster."

*A **Document Imaging System**.* Such a system would be used to electronically store and retrieve scanned images of paper documents (e.g., payment reconciliations received from insurance companies). The system would cost $2,800,000 but would save the organization $1,800,000 per year (or $9,000,000 over the life of the system) due to reduced labor spent looking for paper documents and reduced write-offs that occur because the paper cannot be located.

*An **e-Procurement System**.* This would enable users to order supplies, ensure that the ordering person had the authority to purchase supplies, transmit the order to the supplier and track the receipt of the supplies. Data from this system could be used to support the standardization of supplies. Such standardization might save $500,000 to $3,000,000 per year. The range of savings depends upon physician willingness to standardize. The system would cost $2,500,000.

These proposals (real ones from Partners Healthcare) reflect the diversity of value, ranging from "better disaster response" to a clear financial return (document imaging) to a return with such wide range that it could be a great investment (if the return actually was $3,000,000 per year) or a terrible investment (if the return was only $500,000 per year).

A Single IT Investment Can Have a Diverse Value Proposition

Picture Archival and Communication Systems (PACS) are used to store radiology (and other) images, support interpretation of the image, and distribute the information to the physician providing direct patient care. A PACS can

• Reduce the costs of radiology film and the need for film librarians.

- Improve service to the referring physician delivering care through improved access to images.
- Enable a productivity improvement for the radiologists and the physicians delivering care (both reduce the time they spend looking for images).
- Enable revenue generation if the organization used the PACS to offer radiology services to physician groups in the community.

   A single IT investment can promise diverse value.

Different IT Investment Objectives Have Different Value Assessment Techniques

The return on investment (ROI) is commonly used to evaluate IT proposals. While this approach is not always wrong, neither is it always right.

According to Quinn,[4] there are six categories of IT investments reflecting different objectives. The techniques used to assess IT investments should vary by the type of objective that the IT investment intends to support. One technique does not fit all IT investments.

Infrastructure. IT investments can be infrastructure that enables other investments or applications to be implemented and deliver desired capabilities. Examples of infrastructure include data communication networks, personal computers, and clinical data repositories. A delivery system-wide network enables one to implement applications to consolidate clinical laboratories, establish organization-wide electronic mail and share patient health data between providers.

It is difficult to quantitatively assess the impact or value of infrastructure for several reasons:

- They enable other applications. Without those applications, infrastructure has no value. Hence, infrastructure value is indirect and depends upon application value.
- The ability to allocate infrastructure value across applications is difficult. Of the millions of dollars invested in a data communication network, how much of that investment can be allocated to the cost of delivery system-wide electronic medical records may be difficult or impossible to determine.
- A good IT infrastructure is often determined by its agility, potency and ability to facilitate integration of applications. It is very difficult to assign return on investment numbers or any meaningful "value" number to some of these characteristics. What is the value of being able to, because of agility, speed up the time it takes to develop and enhance applications?

Information system infrastructure is as hard to evaluate as other organizational "infrastructure" such as having talented, educated staff. As with other infrastructure

- Evaluation is often instinctive and experientially based.
- In general, under-investing can severely limit the organization.
- To the degree possible, investment decisions between alternatives should be assessed based upon their ability to achieve agreed upon goals. These goals may be complex to quantify in terms of dollars. Example goals include moving images across the system, high availability of applications and rapid application development.

Mandates. Information system investment may be necessary because of mandated initiatives. Examples of mandated initiatives might include reports of quality data to accrediting organizations, required changes in billing formats or compliance with the Health Insurance Portability and Accountability Act (HIPAA).

Assessing these initiatives is generally approached by identifying the alternative that is the least expensive and the quickest to implement, while achieving some level of compliance.

Cost Reduction. Information system investments directed to cost reduction are generally highly amenable to ROI and other quantifiable dollar impact analyses. The ability to conduct a quantifiable ROI analysis is rarely the question. The ability of management to effect the predicted cost reduction or avoidance is often a far more germane question.

Specific New Products and Services. IT can be critical to the development of new products and services. At times, the information system delivers the new service or is itself the product. Examples of information system-based new services include bank cash management programs and credit card/airline mileage linkage programs. In healthcare, a new service may be Web access, by patients, to guidelines and consumer oriented medical textbooks.

One can quantifiably assess the opportunities in terms of return for some of these new products and services. These assessments include analyses of potential revenues, either directly from the service or service-induced utilization of other products and services. A ROI analysis will need to be supplemented, for example, by techniques such as sensitivity analyses of consumer response.

The value of the investment usually has a speculative component. This component includes customer utilization, competitor response and impact on related businesses.

Quality Improvement. Information system investments are often directed to improving the quality of service or medical care. These investments may intend to reduce waiting times, improve the ability of physicians to locate information, improve treatment outcomes or reduce errors in treatment.

Evaluation of such initiatives, while quantifiable, is generally done in terms of service parameters that are believed to be important measures of service performance. These parameters can be measures of aspects of organizational processes that customers use to judge the organization, for example, waiting times in the physician's office or medication error rates.

A quantifiable dollar outcome of service or care quality improvement can be very hard to predict. Service quality is often necessary to protect current business and the effect of a failure to continuously improve service or medical care can be tough to assess.

Major Strategic Initiative. Strategic initiatives in IT are intended to significantly change the competitive position of the organization or redefine the core nature of the enterprise. In healthcare it is rare that IT is the centerpiece of redefinition of the organization. However, other industries have attempted IT-centric transformations. Amazon.com is an effort to transform retailing. Schwab.com is an undertaking intended to redefine the brokerage industry through the use of the Web.

There can be an ROI core or component to these analyses. However, accurately assessing the ROI of these initiatives and related IT costs can be very problematic. Several factors contribute to this difficulty:

- The initiatives usually recast the company's markets and its roles. The outcome of the recasting, while visionary, can be difficult to see with clarity and certainty.
- The recasting is evolutionary; the organization learns and alters itself as it progresses over what are often lengthy periods of times. It is difficult to be prescriptive about this evolutionary process.
- Market and competitor response can be hard to predict.

Summary

IT is a powerful and diverse tool. It can be applied in a wide range of situations and, as a result, is capable of delivering a wide range of value. Organizations must understand this observation and adapt their evaluation strategies accordingly.

There are times when the ROI is the appropriate investment analysis technique. If a set of investments, including the IT component, is intended to reduce clerical staff, an ROI can be calculated. However, there are times when the ROI is clearly inappropriate. What is the ROI of electronic mail or word processing? One could calculate the ROI but it is hard to imagine an organization basing its investment decision on that analysis.

Would an ROI analysis have captured the strategic value of Internet-based retail applications such as Amazon.com or the value of automated teller machines? Few strategic IT investments have impacts that are fully captured upfront by an ROI. Moreover, the strategic impact is rarely fully understood until years after the investment. Whatever ROI analysis might have been done would have invariably been wrong or highly speculative.

WHY THE IT INVESTMENT FAILS TO DELIVER RETURNS

Despite the complexity and diversity of IT value, organizations do make investment decisions and do implement IT-enabled business initiatives, often in the form of new applications. However, too often management becomes concerned that IT investments have become simply IT expenses. The intended value seems to have disappeared or is a pale shadow of organizational expectations. Why does this happen?

Several reasons for value dilution are listed below and then discussed in more detail.

- A clear linkage is not established between organizational strategy, process redesign and IT investments.
- The wrong question is asked (or, no one understood what the users really needed or worse, the users did not want the solution).
- Goals are not stated (or the expected business benefits are not understood).
- An inappropriate solution is selected.
- Outcomes are not properly managed.
- Project management is mangled, or far less frequently, there is a technical failure in the implementation.

Linkage Failures

The linkage between organizational strategy and the IT strategy can be weak, incomplete or nonexistent. At times, the organizational strategy is troubled. Even if the IT organization is executing well, it may be working on the wrong things or trying to support a flawed overall organizational strategy.

Linkage failures can occur for several reasons:
- The organizational strategy is no more than a slogan or a buzzword, having the depth of a bumper sticker, which makes any investment towards it ill considered.
- IT leadership thinks it understands the business strategy but it does not, resulting in an implementation of an IT version of the strategy rather than the organization's version.
- For a variety of different reasons, the strategists will not engage in the IT discussion, forcing the IT leadership to be mind readers.
- The linkage is superficial, for example, "Patient care systems can reduce nursing labor costs but we have not thought through how that will happen."
- The IT strategy conversation is separated from the normal strategy conversation (for example, an IT Steering Committee with the wrong composition of members), reducing the likelihood of alignment.
- The organizational strategy evolves faster than IT can respond, or conversely, IT applications evolve faster than the organization culture can effectively respond, witnessed by the number of failures of CPOE attempts.
- Even if the IT investment aligns with an organizational strategic goal, if appropriate business process redesign does not exist to accommodate the enabling technology, there may be little benefit realized from the investment.

Asking the Wrong Question

It should be rare that one asks the question, "What is the ROI of a computer system?"

This question makes as much sense as the question "What is the ROI of a chain saw?" If one wants to make a dress, a chain saw is a waste of money. If one wants to cut down some trees, one can begin to think about the return of a chain saw investment and compare that investment to one in an ax. If the chain saw were to be used by one's 10-year-old child, the investment might be ill advised. If the chain saw were to be used by a skilled lumberjack, the investment might be worth it.

One can only determine the ROI, or an investment in any tool, if one knows the task to be performed and the skill level of the participants who are to perform the task. Moreover, a positive ROI is not an inherent property of an IT investment. Once implemented, no computer genie arrives, waves his wand, and magically produces the return. One has to manage a return into existence.

Hence, instead of asking, "What is the ROI of a computer system?" one should ask a series of questions such as:
- What are the steps and investments, including IT, that we need to take or make in order to achieve our goals?
- Which "business" manager owns the achievement of these goals? Do they have our confidence?
- Does the cost, risk and timeframe for the implementation of the set of investments, including the IT investment, seem appropriate given our goals?
- Have we assessed the tradeoffs and opportunity costs?
- Are we comfortable with our ability to execute?

Failure to State Goals

IT proposals are often accompanied by statements about the positive contributions that the investment will make to organizational performance. But the proposals are not always accompanied by specific numeric goals for this improvement. If we intend to reduce medical errors, will we reduce errors by 50% or 80% or some other number? If we intend to reduce claims denials, will we reduce them to 5% or 2%, and how much revenue will be realized as a result of reducing these denials?

Failure to specify explicit numeric goals can create three fundamental value problems:

- We may not know how well we perform now. If we do not know our current error rate or denial rate, it is hard to believe that we have studied the problem well enough to be fairly sure that an IT investment will help achieve the desired gains. The IT proposal sounds more like a guess of what is needed.
- We may never know whether we got the desired value or not. If we do not state a goal, we will never know whether the 20% reduction in errors is as far as we can go or whether we are half way to our desired goal. We do not know whether we should continue to work on the error problem or whether we should move on to the next performance issue.
- It will be difficult to hold someone accountable for performance improvement if we are unable to track how well he or she is doing.

Failure to Manage Outcomes

Related to the above, we often fail to manage the outcome into existence. Once the project is approved and the system is up, management goes off to the next challenge seemingly unaware that the real work of value realization has just begun.

Figure 4-1 depicts the reduction in days in accounts receivable (AR) at a Partners physician practice. During the interval of time depicted, a new practice management system was implemented. One does not see a precipitous decline in days in AR in the time immediately following the implementation. One does see a progressive improvement in days in AR because someone was managing that improvement. The new system was implemented in the second quarter of 1997.

It is very important to have business metrics defined up front so that an organization can measure its performance compared to its plan. The business unit sponsor of the IT-enabled business initiative should be required to supply a series of metrics to measure processes impacted by the IT solution before and after the implementation. The metrics are not necessarily IT-related (up-time, for example), but are business process-related. Patient waiting time, radiology exam turnaround time, or nursing turnover represent some examples.

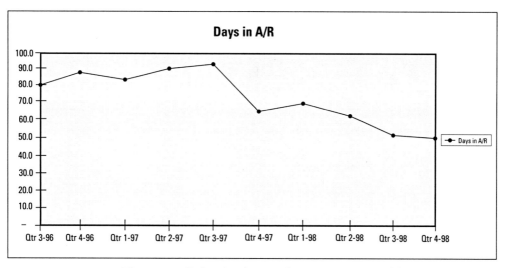

Figure 4-1. Reduction in Days in Accounts Receivable

Ill-Defined Solutions

At times the IT discussion of a new application succumbs to advanced states of technical arousal. Project participants become overwhelmed by the prospect of using sexy new technology and state-of-the-art gizmos and lose their senses and understanding of why they are having this discussion in the first place. Sexiness and state-of-the-art-ness become the criteria for making system decisions.

In addition, the comparison of two alternative vendor products can get lost in the features beauty contest. One product out-features another. The discussion devolves into a features war.

Both sexiness and features have their place in the system selection decision. However, they are secondary to the discussion that centers on the capabilities needed to affect specific performance goals. Sexiness and features can be irrelevant to the performance improvement discussion. Further, system selection decisions should also be based on an understanding of how much an organization is willing to modify its business processes to accommodate the design and workflow of the various alternative systems. Unless an organization is a huge academic medical center with hundreds of programmers at its disposal, the organization should buy an application from a vendor. The various applications are designed differently, and their workflow is different. Trying to modify one of them to do things the way an organization has always done them is tantamount to pounding the square peg into a round hole. To get the maximum value from the investment, an organization has to know how each of the vendors accomplishes the automation of the processes that it is trying to improve and pick the one that most closely fits the organization's willingness and capability to change.

Mangled Project Management

One guaranteed way to reduce value is to mangle the management of the implementation project. Implementation failures or significant budget and timetable overruns or really unhappy users all dilute value.

Projects become mangled for many reasons, including:
- Project scope is poorly defined.
- Accountability is unclear.
- The project participants are marginally skilled.
- The magnitude of the task is underestimated.
- Users feel like victims rather than participants.
- All of the world has a vote and can vote at any time.

Studies on IT Value Achievement

A study by Quinn[4] found that the major contributors to failure to achieve a solid return on IT investments were:
- A suboptimal organizational strategy or organizational assessment of its competitive environment. Insufficient return occurs because the overall strategy is wrong.
- The strategy is fine but the associated IT capabilities are not defined appropriately. The information system, if it is solving a problem, is solving the wrong problem.
- Failure to identify and draw together well all investments and initiatives necessary to carry out the organization's plans. The IT investment falters because other changes, such as reorganization or re-engineering, fail to occur.
- Failure to execute the plan well. Poor planning or less than stellar management can diminish the return from any investment.

Value can be diluted by factors outside of the organization's control. Weill[5] noted that the more strategic the IT investment the more its value can be diluted. An IT investment directed to increasing market share can have its value diluted by non-IT decisions and events (for example, pricing decisions), the actions of competitors and the reaction of customers. IT investments which are less strategic but have business value (for example, improving nursing productivity), can also be diluted by factors outside of the control of management (for example, shortages of nursing staff). The value of an IT investment directed towards improving the characteristics of the infrastructure can be diluted by factors outside the control of the IT organization, for example, unanticipated technology immaturity or business difficulties confronting a vendor.

Summary

A wide range of factors can diminish IT value. Value dilution can occur well before the project even starts. For an organization to ensure consistent value delivery it must manage an array of management processes and factors, strategic IT planning, the composition of its leadership, its budget processes, and its project management approaches.

ACHIEVING SUSTAINED, HIGH LEVELS OF IT-ENABLED VALUE

Several studies (McKenney et al,[6] Ross et al,[7] Sambamurthy et al,[8] and Weill and Broadbent[5]) have examined organizations that have achieved very high levels of IT-enabled value over the course of many years, often decades. Organizations that were studied include American Airlines, Bank of America, Federal Express and the former American Hospital Supply.

The studies suggest that organizations that aspire to high levels of effectiveness and innovation in their application of IT must take steps to ensure that the core capacity of the organization to achieve value is developed. The development of this capacity is a different challenge than effecting specific opportunities to use IT in the course of improving operations or enhancing management decision-making.

As an analogy, a runner's training, injury management and diet are designed to ensure his or her core capacity to run a marathon. This capacity development is different from the approach to running a specific marathon that must consider the nature of the course, the competing runners and the weather.

While having somewhat different conclusions (resulting to a degree from somewhat different study questions), the four studies have much in common regarding capacity development.

Individuals and Leadership Matter

It is critical that the organization possess talented, skilled and experienced individuals. These individuals will occupy a variety of roles: CEO, CFO, CIO, IT staff and user middle management. These individuals must be strong contributors. While such an observation may seem trite, too often organizations, dazzled by the technology or the glorified experiences of others, embark upon technology crusades and substantive investments for which they have insufficient talent to effect well.

Leadership in these organizations was essential. This leadership was needed on the part of organizational senior management, the CFO, the CIO and the project team. It understood the vision, communicated the vision, was able to recruit and motivate a team, and had the staying power to see the achievement of value through several years of work, disappointments, setbacks and political problems along the way.

Relationships Are Critical

In addition to strong individual players, the team must be strong. There are critical roles among senior executives, IT executives, and project team members that must be filled by highly competent individuals. In addition, great chemistry must exist between the individuals in the distinct roles. Substituting team members, while perhaps involving a replacement by an equally strong individual, can diminish the team. This is true in IT effectiveness just as it is true in sports. Political turbulence diminished the ability to develop a healthy set of relationships between organizational players.

Technology and Technical Infrastructure Both Enables and Hinders

New technologies can provide new opportunities for organizations to embark upon major improvements of their activities. This implies that, while the CIO must have superior business and clinical understanding, he or she must also have superior understanding of the technology. This should not imply that the CIO can rewrite operating systems as well as the best system programmers, but it does mean that the CIO has superior understanding of the maturity, capabilities and possible evolutions of IT. Several major achievements of value occurred because the IT group was able to identify and adopt an emerging technology that made a significant contribution to addressing a current organizational challenge.

The studies stress the importance of well-developed technical architecture. Great architecture matters. Possessing state of the art technology can be far less important than a well-integrated, reliable and supportable set of IT.

The Organization Must Encourage Innovation

The organization's (and the IT organization's) culture and leadership must encourage innovation and experimentation. This encouragement needs to be practical and goal directed. There must be a real business problem, crisis or opportunity, and the project will need budgets, political protection and deliverables.

Significant Value Achievement Takes Time

Achieving exceptional gains in performance takes time and a lot of work (Collins[9]). Organizations often took five to seven years for major initiatives to fully mature and the value to be seen. The applications and designs proceed through phases, for example, conception, analysis, piloting and rollout that are as normative as the passage from childhood to maturity. Major organizational improvements, like the maturation of a human being, will see some variation in the timing, depth and success at moving through phases.

Evaluation of IT Opportunities Must Be Thoughtful

The IT initiatives studied were analyzed and studied thoroughly. Nonetheless, the organizations engaged in these initiatives understood that a large element of vision, management instinct and "feel" often guided the decision to initiate investment and continue investment. An organization that has had more experience with IT and more successful experiences will be more effective in the evaluation (and execution) of IT-enabled business initiatives.

Initiatives Were Based on Processes, Data, and Differentiation

All of these organizations had fundamental understandings of the current limitations of the organization's processes, services, market position and management reporting. The initiatives studied were directed to focus on core elements:

- Significant leveraging of organizational processes, for example, revenue cycle, test and procedure ordering or patient access to care;
- Expanding and capitalizing upon the ability to gather critical data, for example, referral patterns and care quality; and/or
- Achieving a high level of organizational differentiation, for example, low cost care delivery or distinctive high quality care delivery.

Often an initiative pursued all three simultaneously. At times the organization evolved from one element to another as the competition responded and/or it saw new leverage points.

Strong "IT Asset"

Very competent IT staff, well-designed IT governance and decision-making mechanisms, well-crafted architecture and superb IT project management were critical attributes for achieving sustained value.

Strong Alignment of IT Strategy and Organizational Strategy

This finding of alignment in the studies was explored, in depth, by Earl[10] in a study of organizations in England that had a history of IT excellence. Earl found that their IT planning processes had several characteristics.

- IT planning, and the strategic discussion of IT, occurred as an integral part of organizational strategic planning processes and management discussions. In these organizations, management did not think of separating out an IT discussion during the course of strategy development, any more than they would run a separate finance or human resources planning process. IT planning was an unseverable, intertwined component of the normal management conversation. These organizations did not have a separate IT steering committee.

- Often IT planning processes start in one month every year and are completed, for example, three months later. In the studied organizations, the IT planning and strategy conversation went on continuously. This does not mean that an organization does not have to have a temporally de-marked process designed to form a budget every year. Rather, it means that IT planning is a continuous process reflecting the continuous change in the environment and organizational plans and strategies.

- IT planning involved shared decision-making and shared learning between IT and the organization. IT leadership informed organizational leadership of the potential contribution of new technologies and constraints of current technologies. Organizational leadership ensured that IT leadership understood the business plans and strategies and constraints. The IT budget and annual tactical plan resulted from a shared analyses and set of conclusions.

- The IT plan emphasized themes. A provider organization may have themes of improving care quality, reducing costs and integrating the delivery system. During the course of any given year, it will have initiatives that are intended to advance the organization along these themes. The mixture of initiatives will change from year to year but the themes endure over the course of many years.

  Themes, such as care improvement, help organizations understand the need for foundation initiatives such as the establishment of a group to measure care quality or the standardization on common vocabularies for clinical data. Themes provide a basis for crafting technical architecture; for example, infrastructure reliability and performance become exceptionally important if significant, multi-year investments will be made in systems to be used directly by care providers.

Summary

Achieving IT-enabled value over the course of many projects and many years requires a "core IT capacity." This capacity is diverse and includes talented people, great working relationships, organizational thoughtfulness and mature IT alignment. This capacity is probably not materially different from the core capacity to effect organizational excellence in general.

It may be more important for an organization to work on improving its core capacity than it is to work on any specific IT application. One might be able to get through one marathon without developing the capacity to run marathons but it is unlikely that one will be able to run several marathons. Unfortunately, it is not common to see, in an organization's IT plan for the year, a discussion centered on improving core IT capacity.

INCREASING THE DELIVERY OF IT VALUE

IT value is complex and diverse. Several factors can diminish the realization of IT value. Organizations should also recognize that steps can be taken to develop the core ability to deliver IT value over the course of many projects and several years. In bringing closure to this chapter, what overall actions should organizations take to increase the returns from IT investments (Dragoon[11])?

Make Sure Homework Is Done

IT investment decisions are often made based on proposals that are not resting on a solid ground. In such instances, the proposers have not done their homework and hence the risk of a suboptimal return has been elevated.

Clearly the track record of the investment proposer has a significant influence on the likelihood of a favorable investment decision being made and the resulting investment delivering value. However, regardless of track record, IT-enabled business initiative proposals should enable the audience to respond with a strong "yes" to each of the following questions.

- Is it clear how the plan advances the organization's strategy?
- Is it clear how care will improve, costs will be reduced or service will be improved? Are the measures of current performance and expected improvement well researched and realistic? Have the related changes in operations, workflow and organization been defined?
- Is the senior leadership, whose areas are the focus of the IT plan, clearly supportive and could they give the presentation?
- Are the resource requirements well understood and convincingly presented? Have these requirements been compared to those experienced by other organizations undertaking similar initiatives?
- Have the investment risks been identified and is there an approach to addressing these risks?
- Are the right people assigned to the project, has their time been freed up, and are they well organized?

A negative answer, or perhaps an "equivocal yes" to any of these questions, should lead one to believe that the discussion is perhaps focusing on an expense rather than an investment.

Use Techniques for Comparing Different Types of Value

Given the diversity of value, it is very challenging to compare different IT proposals that have different value propositions. How does one compare a proposal that promises to increase revenue and improve collaboration with one that offers improved compliance, faster turnaround times and reduced supply costs?

At the end of the day, judgment is used to choose one proposal over another. Managers review the various proposals and their value statements and make choices based on their sense of organizational priorities, available monies and the likelihood that the value will be seen.

These judgments can be aided by the development of a scoring approach that helps to develop a common "metric" across proposals. For example, the organization can decide to score each proposal according to how well it meets the following criteria:

- Revenue impact
- Cost reduction
- Patient/customer satisfaction
- Quality of work life
- Quality of care
- Regulatory compliance
- Potential learning value

Each proposal is assigned a score, for each criterion, ranging from 5 (significant contribution to the criterion) to 1 (minimal or no contribution). The scores are totaled and, in theory, one picks those proposals with the highest aggregate scores. In practice such scoring can be very helpful in sorting through complex and diverse value propositions:

- Scoring forces the leadership team to discuss why different members of the team used different scores, for example, why someone assigned a score of 2 for revenue impact while someone else assigned a 4? Resolving these different perceptions clarifies any misunderstandings of proposal objectives and helps the team arrive at a consensus regarding the project.
- Scoring means that the leadership team will have to defend a decision to not fund a project with a high score or fund one with a low score. For example, why does everyone favor of this project if it has such a low score?

The organization can decide which criteria to use and which will not be used. Some organizations give different criteria different weights, e.g., reducing costs is twice as important as improving organizational learning. The resulting scores are not binding but they can be helpful in arriving at an organizational decision about which projects will be approved and what value is being sought.

Increase Accountability for Investment Results

Few meaningful organization initiatives are accomplished without establishing appropriate accountability for results. Accountability for IT investment results can be improved by taking two major steps during the budget process.

First, during the budget request, the business owner of the IT investment should defend the investment. For example, the head of clinical laboratories should defend the request for a new laboratory system and the head of nursing should defend the need for a new nursing system. The IT staff will need to work with the business owner to define IT costs, establish likely implementation timeframes and sort through application alternatives.

IT should prepare the budget needed to support existing applications and infrastructure. And the CIO should defend new infrastructure initiatives, such as improved network security or the purchase of new storage technologies. However, the IT staff should never defend an application investment.

Second, the presentation of these projects should occur as part of the overall organizational capital and operating budget development process and meetings; there is no separate track for IT discussions. In other words, budget requests for new IT applications are reviewed in the same conversation that discusses budget requests for new clinical services diagnostic equipment.

These two steps mean that a sponsor, for example, a clinical vice president, will defend "his" IT request in front of "his" colleagues. The sponsor will determine whether to present the IT proposal or some other, perhaps non-IT, proposal.

The sponsor and his or her colleagues know that if the IT proposal is approved there will be less money available for other initiatives. This forces the defender to be convinced of the value, have a good understanding of how to achieve the value and be committed to achieving the value. The defender also knows that the value being promised must be delivered or their credibility, during budget discussions next year, will be diminished. Accountability must be accompanied by consequences.

Examine IT Investments as a Portfolio

The presentation and discussion of IT project funding decisions should occur in a forum that routinely reviews these requests. The consistency of using the same forum enables the forum participants to develop a seasoned understanding of good versus not so good proposals since they will see many proposals over the course of time. And the forum can compare and contrast proposals as it decides which ones should be approved. A manager might wonder, with good reason, "If I approve this proposal, does that mean that we won't have resources for another project that I might like even better?" Examining as many proposals together as possible enables the organization to take a portfolio view of its potential investments.

An example portfolio is presented in Figure 4-2. The size of the bubble reflects that magnitude of the IT investment. The axes are labeled reward (the size of the expected value) and risk (the relative risk that the project will not deliver the value). Other axes can be used. One often sees an axis with one row labeled "support of operations" and the other labeled "support strategic initiatives."

Diagrams such as these serve several functions:

- They enable the leadership to have "one piece of paper" that summarizes their IT activity and allows them to consider a new request in the context of prior commitments.
- They help to ensure that the portfolio does not become too imbalanced. Imbalance can occur when the projects cluster in one quadrant or, for example, indicate that the vast majority of IT initiatives carry high risk.
- The diagram can help to ensure that the approved projects cover an appropriate spectrum of organizational needs; for example, there are projects that are directed to revenue cycle improvement and operational improvement and patient safety.

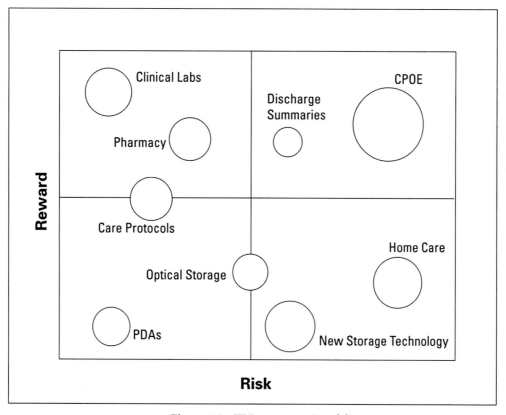

Figure 4-2. IT Investment Portfolio

Conduct Post-Implementation Audits

Rarely do organizations revisit their IT investments to determine if the promised value was actually achieved. Organizations believe that, once the implementation settles down, value will have been automatically achieved. This is unlikely.

Post-implementation audits should be conducted to identify value achievement progress and steps still needed to achieve maximum gain. An organization can decide to audit two to four systems each year and select systems that have been "live" for at least six months. During the course of the audit meeting, five questions can be asked:

- What were the goals of the investment that were expected at the time the project was approved?
- How close have we come to achieving our original goals?
- What do we need to do to close the goal gap?
- How much have we invested in the implementation of the system and how does that compare to our original budget?
- If we had to implement this system again, what would we do differently?
  Post-implementation audits assist value achievement by:
- Signaling leadership interest in ensuring the delivery of results.
- Identifying steps that still need to be taken to ensure value.
- Supporting organizational learning about IT value realization.
- Reinforcing accountability for results.

Celebrate Value Achievement

Business value should be celebrated. Organizations usually hold parties shortly after applications "go live." These parties are appropriate; a lot of people worked very hard to get the system up and running and used.

However, up and running and used does not mean that value has been delivered. In addition to go-live parties, organizations should consider business value parties; celebrations conducted once the value has been achieved, e.g., a party that celebrates the achievement of service improvement goals.

Go-live parties risk sending an inappropriate signal that implementation is the end point of the IT initiative.

Leverage Organizational Governance

The creation of an IT subcommittee of the board can enhance organizational efforts to achieve value from their IT investments. At times, the leadership of organizations are uncomfortable with some or all of the IT conversation. They may not understand why infrastructure is so expensive, or why large implementations can take so long and cost so much. The creation of a subcommittee that has members more experienced with these discussions can help to ensure that hard questions are being asked and that the answers are sound.

The leadership should not believe that such a subcommittee gets them off the hook for having to deal with IT issues. Rather the committee should be viewed as a way for the leadership to continue their efforts to become more knowledgeable and comfortable with the IT conversation.

Shorten the Cycle of Deliverables

When possible, projects should have short deliverable cycles. In other words, rather than waiting 12 months or 18 months for the organization to see the first fruits of its application system implementation labors, efforts should be made to deliver a sequence of smaller implementations.

This shortening can take the form of pilots of an application in a subset of the organization followed by a staged rollout. Another possibility would be the serial implementation of 25% of the eventual 100% of application features.

It is not always possible to have pilots, staged rollouts, or the implementation of a portion of the application. However, shortened deliverable cycles enable the organization to achieve some value earlier rather than later. In addition, they support organizational learning about what system capabilities are really important versus those that were thought to be important, facilitate the development of re-engineered operational processes, and create the appearance (not to be under estimated) of more value delivery.

Benchmark Value

Organizations should benchmark their performance with their peers. These benchmarks can focus on process performance (e.g., days in accounts receivables or average time to get an appointment). An important aspect of these value benchmarks is the identification of critical IT application capabilities and related operational changes that enabled the achievement of superior results.

This understanding of how other organizations achieved superior IT-enabled performance guides organizational efforts to continuously achieve as much value as possible from their IT investments.

Summary

One cannot expect to realize the business value of an IT investment unless one aligns the following (Figure 4-3):

- The forces pressing on the organization (industry, economic, regulatory, environmental, sociological, technological, and political drivers);
- The organization's business vision and goals;
- The decisions that the organization must make to achieve its vision and goals; and
- The process changes that will bring those decisions to life.

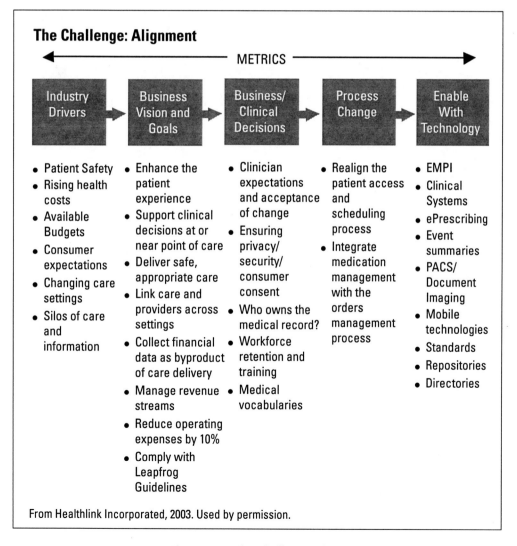

Figure 4-3. The Challenge: Alignment

Achieving the alignment is difficult in the best of circumstances, but is impossible if the proper governance is not in place to manage the alignment and if business metrics are not adopted to measure the performance of the redesigned, IT-enabled processes.

Achieving value from IT investments is hard, ongoing work. However, it does not involve magic or require that organizational leadership learn new techniques. Asking hard questions, holding people accountable and reviewing investment performance are attributes of good management regardless of whether the topic is IT, finance or patient care.

No new management techniques are required to evaluate IT plans, proposals and progress. Leadership is often asked to make decisions that involve strategic hunches (a strategy to develop a continuum of care), where they may have limited domain knowledge (new surgical modalities) and where the value is fuzzy (improved morale).

Organizational leadership should treat IT investments no differently than these other types of investments; if leadership does not understand, believe or trust the proposal or proponent, the investment should not be approved. And if leadership does not understand the CIO, it is the CIO's fault.

The IT investment/value challenge plagues all industries. This is not a problem peculiar to healthcare. The challenge has existed for 40 years, ever since organizations began to spend money on big mainframes. This challenge is complex and persistent and will not be able to be resolved completely. Nevertheless, organizational leadership should believe that it can become better at dealing with it.

John P. Glaser, PhD, FCHIME, FHIMSS, is Vice-President and Chief Information Officer, Partners HealthCare System, Inc. Dr. Glaser was the founding chairman of College of Healthcare Information Management Executives (CHIME) and is past chair of the HIMSS. He is a fellow of HIMSS, CHIME and the American College of Medical Informatics. He has been awarded the John Gall Award for Healthcare CIO of the Year. CHIME has established a scholarship in Dr. Glaser's name. He was a recipient of CIO Magazine's 20/20 Vision Award. His organization, Partners HealthCare, has received several industry awards for its effective and innovative use of information technology. Dr. Glaser is on the editorial boards of CIO Magazine, Healthcare Informatics, Journal of Biomedical Informatics, and Journal of Healthcare Information Management. He has published over 80 articles and two books on the strategic application of information technology in healthcare. He holds a PhD in healthcare information systems from the University of Minnesota.

David E. Garets, FHIMSS, is President and CEO of HIMSS Analytics. With 27 years of experience in information technology, Mr. Garets joined HIMSS Analytics in 2004 from Healthlink Incorporated where he was Executive Vice President. Prior to that, he was Group Vice President, Healthcare Industry Research and Advisory Services at Gartner, Inc. Before joining Gartner in 1998, Mr. Garets was with First Consulting Group where he was Senior Manager in Emerging Practices and also served as CIO of Magic Valley Regional Medical Center in Twin Falls, Idaho, for five years. He was a course director and served on the faculties of the CHIME Information Management Executive Courses for 11 years. Mr. Garets serves on the editorial advisory boards of seven health care information technology journals and magazines and is a HIMSS Fellow. He was Chair of the HIMSS Board of Directors for 2003–2004.

References

1. Glaser J: Analyzing Information Technology Value. *Healthcare Financial Management.* March 2003; 98–104.
2. Wang S, et al: A Cost-Benefit Analysis of the Electronic Medical Record in Primary Care. *American Journal of Medicine.* 2003; 114; 397–403.
3. Bates D, et al: Effect of Computerized Physician Order Entry and a Team Intervention on Prevention of Serious Medication Errors. *JAMA.* 1998; 280(15); 1311–1316.
4. Quinn JB, et al: *Information Technology in the Service Society.* Washington DC: National Academy Press; 1994.
5. Weill P, Broadbent M: *Leveraging the New Infrastructure.* Boston: Harvard Business School Press; 1998.
6. McKenney J, Copeland D, Mason R: *Waves of Change: Business Evolution Through Information Technology.* Boston, MA: Harvard Business School Press; 1995.
7. Ross J, Beath C, Goodhue D: Develop Long-Term Competitiveness through IT Assets. *Sloan Management Review.* 1996; 38(1); 31–42.
8. Sambamurthy V, Zmud R: *Information Technology and Innovation: Strategies for Success.* Morristown, NJ: Financial Executives Research Foundation; 1996.
9. Collins J: *Good to Great.* New York, NY: HarperCollins; 2001.
10. Earl M: Experiences in Strategic IT Planning. *MIS Quarterly.* 1993; 17(1); 1–24.
11. Dragoon A: Deciding Factors. *CIO Magazine.* Aug 15, 2003; 49–59.

Bibliography

Arloto P, Oakes J: *Return on Investment: Maximizing the Value of Healthcare Information Technology.* Chicago, IL: Healthcare Information and Management Systems Society; 2003.

Glaser J: Why Does an IT Investment Fail to Deliver Returns? *Healthcare Financial Management.* Apr 2003; 114–118.

Glaser J: When IT Excellence Goes the Distance. *Healthcare Financial Management.* Sep 2003; 102–106.

Glaser J, DeBor G, Stuntz L: The New England Healthcare EDI Network. *Journal of Healthcare Information Management* (in press).

Glaser J: *The Strategic Application of Information Technology in Healthcare Organizations. Second Edition.* San Francisco, CA: Jossey-Bass; 2002.

CHAPTER 5

Where's the Beef? Part 2: Assessing an IT Organization's Performance

Terence T. Cunningham, III, MHA, FACHE, and
Stephanie L. Reel, MBA

During a hallway conversation, the Chief Medical Officer complained to Sam Weatherspoon about the time it took IS to implement systems as well as the fact that the physicians viewed the ones that were delivered as decidedly mediocre. Moreover, the CMO had attended a conference last week and heard a CIO from the east coast talk about this incredible set of applications that had been implemented in an amazingly short period of time. The question the CMO asked Sam was, "Why can't our IS group do what the speaker's organization appeared to have done?"

Sam wasn't sure how to respond. His previous discussions with the Ingalls' CIO had led him to be quite empathetic to the difficulty of implementing complex applications and the challenges of dealing with vendors. Nonetheless, was the Ingalls IS group mediocre at best?

As the hospital CEO, Sam Witherspoon is determined to provide all of his departments, including IT, with effective leadership. Among the critical functions he must perform is to gain an understanding of what is happening in IT. He must also determine how IT planning activities and operations should be assessed. In addition, Sam must define how he can partner with the CIO and senior IT leadership to maximize the value derived from the investment of scarce healthcare dollars into information technologies.

Sam readily admits that he is puzzled by much of the IT jargon and is awed by the mysterious pieces of computer equipment that IT maintains. He does have a general sense, though, of what the clinical staff, administration and others expect from IT. Basically, they want timely, reliable, accurate, user friendly and useful information that can be easily understood and utilized. Achieving this goal is genuinely challenging and will require tremendous coordination, collaboration, and communication at all levels in the organization. Ideally, Sam, together with his CIO and other key staff members, must develop a strong mutual commitment for IT to become credible and highly effective.

Sam also realizes that new organizational models may be in order, requiring different competencies to enhance the IT offerings at his institution. He understands the importance of effective governance and customer-centric service groups across the enterprise as well as within his IT staff. He also understands the value of "disruptive technologies" and will be supportive of the cultural and behavioral changes that his team must endorse. And, of course, Sam wants to ensure that this critical department is not only serving his institution well but is also well positioned for influencing the future from the standpoint of infrastructure as well as innovation.

Sam begins this journey by looking at the most fundamental IT operations while trying to determine, with the CIO, how to best assess IT activities that are serving the hospital well, where value is being realized, and where there are deficits that need attention.

Sam understands the value of external benchmarks and industry best practices. He noted in *Modern Healthcare's* annual survey of IS trends (Figure 5-1) that hospitals were planning to invest for 2003 in IT and system solutions.

Trend	Percentage
Use imaging technologies (e.g., Internet)	53%
Address changes (e.g., HIPAA)	52%
Improve decision support for clinicians	51%
Improve productivity and reduce costs	46%
Improve patient care capabilities	36%
Integrate data bases	29%
Improve patient accounting	19%
Use LANs, respond to consumers, improve benefit of technology, improve ambulatory capabilities (all 15%)	15%
Improve general accounting	11%
Improve managed care	9%

Figure 5-1. Annual Survey of IS Trends in Healthcare (2003)[1]

Sam decides to work with the CIO in designing a set of metrics and parameters that can be quantified to measure current operations. He appreciates the value of measuring performance objectively and in unambiguous ways. He also appreciates the value of collaboration in the healthcare business and agrees that much of the activities of his IT department and his CIO are based upon good communication skills, excellent relationship management techniques, and disciplined planning and development activities.

Sam has collected some of these metrics and has created a series of questions, some of which can be readily presented in a dashboard format that can routinely be updated, reviewed and evaluated. Others may be more subjective.

Sam considers all of these questions and answers to be the blueprint for evaluating the value of his IT organization. He believes that they can serve any CEO as he or she attempts to grasp the fundamental services and values that the IT organization is providing. The questions, which are addressed in this chapter, revolve around **12 topics**

that will help senior management focus on improving the CEO and CIO partnership. The topics include:

1. System availability;
2. System reliability;
3. Usability;
4. Spam and related concerns;
5. Security;
6. Strategic planning;
7. Project management;
8. Staff development;
9. Productivity and cost management;
10. Alternate management and support structures;
11. Vendor management, contract negotiations, and contract management; and
12. Future concerns.

SYSTEM AVAILABILITY

Computer/Systems Uptime

Uptime is a measurement of the time the computer is available for use, in contrast to downtime, when the computer is unavailable. The goal is to have zero unscheduled downtime. The uptime should be measured daily and downtime captured by times of the day and days of the week. Scheduled versus unscheduled downtime should also be recorded. Scheduled downtime should be at times that will be minimally disruptive to patient care delivery.

Computer/Systems Downtime

There are several ways to measure systems downtime. However, the true measurement of downtime is based upon the perception of the end users. If a hardware platform experiences no unscheduled downtime but the end user experiences a problem that prevents access or inappropriately limits access to required applications or critical information (password denial, network performance, workstation failure, etc.), the perception of downtime becomes the reality for the end user.

For this reason, it is important to consider the end-to-end performance of the system, rather than isolated data center metrics. This measurement can provide a challenge for complex organizations, where reliability may depend upon commodity Internet availability, wireless access points, directory services and Web services.

The value of tracking the various forms of access has become meaningful as productivity, safety and security have become critical components of the total environment. Sam's CIO also realizes that the complexity of an environment often contributes to poor performance or unscheduled downtime. This conversation with Sam provides the CIO with an opportunity to lobby for a standards-based approach to the selection, deployment and support of information technologies.

SYSTEM RELIABILITY

Sam also wants to ensure that his leadership team trusts the systems. Therefore, he chooses to focus his next series of questions around the accuracy and timeliness of the information. If Sam's leadership team is searching for quality information and is unable to find it where and when they need it, his CIO may not be providing the level of value that is expected and required in a dynamic health care environment.

Some relevant questions include the following:

- How accurate and timely is information?
- How trusted is it?
- How consistent are the definitions of the information?
- How well understood are the processes and data flows that are producing the information?

An institutional computer system or suite of information systems should provide accurate and consistent data 100% of the time. Consistent values, agreed upon definitions, and timely reporting of data are critical for decision-making. Ideally, the data is real time, or if not, footnoted with an explanation or an "as of" date. Where there may be confusion, footnotes and legends should automatically be provided to explain how information is derived or calculated, and a point of contact listed as a method of obtaining additional clarification of the data.

One example of confusion could result from the mechanisms used to track occupancy levels or census statistics, or even numbers of inpatient or outpatient registrations and visits. Tracking the denominator often inserts ambiguity. Some institutions track occupancy based upon licensed beds, others based upon open or managed beds, and still others based upon staffed beds. Tracking of the midnight census may be a typical metric for some institutions, while others are concerned about the census at 10 a.m., after most discharges have been completed for the day. Although this trivial example can be well explained, lack of a clear definition can create a lack of credibility for the system and the system manager. In fact, confusing data points should be anticipated and explanations provided to enhance accuracy.

Sam also worries that the information may not be appropriately configured to support business decisions. The systems may be available and may contain reliable information, but they may not be adequately integrated to ensure meaningful comparisons or relevant trends. Sam's CIO explains the benefit of data marts and aggregated data warehousing technologies (see Chapter 8 for a more in-depth treatment of this topic).

USABILITY

Sam also realizes that comfort levels vary with IT. Some of the members of the leadership team are perfectly comfortable with wireless, hand-held access, using PDAs and tablets to access and update information. Other team members struggle with e-mail. Sam wants all members of the team to be able to effectively use information. He asks his CIO a series of related questions:

- Are the computer systems user friendly, readily accessible, and easily used where they are needed, and when they are needed?

- Are the tools listed below appropriately and affordably being made available to the users who need them?

Wireless Access/WiFi

Wireless fidelity, or having the ability of wireless connection to laptops on mobile carts, PC notebooks and PDAs with the ability to enter, retrieve and query, regardless of geographic location of the user, are more commonly being adopted in healthcare settings.

Electronic Signature

As the industry embraces a migration to a wireless and paperless environment, systems must provide tracking mechanisms that are auditable. The introduction of rigorous auditing and tracking techniques has promoted a broader acceptance of electronic signatures, allowing for much less reliance on paper. However, until the "tipping point" is reached where paper is no longer the accepted standard, the promised cost reductions or productivity gains that must be achieved to support continued investments will not be realized. Electronic signatures are one of the tools that must be uniformly accepted to ensure compliance, without continued commitment to paper.

Biometrics

Access and authentication technologies have evolved and are continuing to evolve, particularly as secure remote access to clinical data is expected and required. Authentication is needed to support medical legal authorization. Retinal or iris scans, facial recognition, voice recognition, unique password and user ID techniques, and fingerprint recognition tools are being more widely adopted and more broadly deployed.

The fundamental approach is intended to permit rapid ease of access, but only to the right person. This approach is intended to encourage the right user to provide something they know (a password), together with something they have (a token or an identification badge), and something they "are" (thumbprint, retinal scan, and the like).

Bar Coding

This 30-year-old technology allows for rapid identification of patients, care providers, locations, supplies, medications, interventions and results that can be entered into a medical record. The technology is now being replaced in many settings with radio frequency identification "tags," commonly abbreviated as RFID. Although still unacceptably expensive for low cost items, pilot projects are underway to support equipment tracking and limited medication management.[2]

Single Sign-on and/or Split Screen Technology

Technologies and tools are evolving toward more effectively supporting the increasing complexity that is overwhelming the healthcare environment. The presentation layer of information technologies has become a critical component of the quest for simplification of the complexity of the industry. Filtering techniques, smart agents and monitoring tools should allow for the creation of "just in time" and "just for me" presentations of information.

Redundancy, Disaster Recovery, and Business Continuity

As healthcare organizations have come to depend upon applications and technologies to conduct business and care for patients, it has become essential that systems and information are protected against the threat of loss or corruption. Ensuring that systems are appropriately protected and that data is appropriately and routinely copied to other media and stored in remote locations, must be an expectation. Recovery technologies and policies and procedures must be documented and practiced often enough to ensure that a disaster can be adequately addressed. Retrieval techniques, together with the user sponsors, must be tested to ensure that the end-to-end information access and process flow can be replicated upon recovery following an event.

Security and Firewalls

The systems should fully comply with federal legislation under the Health Insurance Portability and Accountability Act (HIPAA). This includes tracking of access and tiered controls so that only pre-identified individuals have access to designated categories of information, with auditable record trails. Physical and logical firewalls, packet filters, and intrusion detection technologies must be implemented, managed and maintained. Policies must be endorsed and enforced to ensure consistent compliance with expectations.

Communication Technologies

Pagers, beepers, e-mail systems and alert systems must be integrated to ensure that patient information can reach the care providers in a timely way. Panic values, or significant changes in a patient's condition, should be communicated to an attending or referring physician as rapidly as possible. Many information systems now support rapid communication techniques to ensure timely notification and reliable tracking of the information flow.

SPAM AND RELATED CONCERNS

Strong technical management is also important to Sam. He wants to be certain that his organization is being protected from waste and inefficiencies as technologies are more broadly deployed. He asks questions about Spam, virus protection, and Web abuse.

Spam

Are technologies in place to protect users from unnecessary and unwanted e-mail or inappropriate information? Is an effective Spam control system in use? Various software systems can screen out unwanted electronic mail to predetermine sensitivity. The system can also record the number of Spam messages received and blocked. User feedback can also determine the amount of the same Spam that is reaching users that can be added to the blocked list.

Virus Protection

Is a dynamic virus protection system in use? Users will quickly detect slowdowns in the system and loss of data and functionality. IT virus systems must remain current to protect against viruses, worms and other destructive electronic programs sent through e-mail. This can accidentally occur when unsuspecting users of the system upload data from outside sources. User feedback will provide this measure.

Web Abuse

Is Web abuse being tracked? Use of the Internet should be encouraged for business-related use. However, abuse of Web access should be discouraged and tracked. For instance, users contacting addresses on lottery results, shopping sites, pornographic sites, and other obvious non-business-related sites can be recorded and the users confronted. There are systems that limit Web access and record the amount of time users access various sites.

SECURITY

While Sam worries about protecting his staff, he also worries about protecting the organization's assets. Security and business assets and the protection of intellectual property are just two examples of Sam's areas of concern. He is also concerned about protecting medical records, employee records, and other private information. He asks his CIO about the security measures that exist to protect this information. Among his questions are the following:

- Are appropriate internal controls in place to protect the institution?
- Are annual software and hardware audits conducted of all purchased and leased items and what corrective actions are being taken?
- Are system controls (problem management, change control, control totals) being regularly audited for compliance purposes?

Underutilized or inappropriately used systems should be routinely evaluated and considered for "sunsetting" or replacement. The elimination of obsolete systems is often ignored and can potentially add to a cost burden or a misuse of unmanaged information. Boutique software systems and some homegrown solutions should be considered for integration into vendor-supplied or otherwise existing generic software.

System interfaces should also be subjected to review to ensure that data controls are in place to protect against inappropriate use or manipulation of information that might be used fraudulently. Internal and external audits of such controls should be incorporated into the institution's annual audit process.

In addition, equipment should also be inventoried, tracked and managed in an institutional asset management system to ensure protection against loss, theft, or mismanagement.

STRATEGIC PLANNING

Sam needs to ensure that the organization takes a long-term view of IT and that the strategy is tightly coupled with the corporate strategy. Because the rate of change is so rapid, the CEO wants to ensure that his CIO has a plan and continuously refreshes it based on business imperatives rather than technology for its own sake. He asks his CIO the following questions to help him understand the IT planning processes:

- Is there a process in place to provide guidance to the IT department as an integral component of the strategic plan?
- Are priorities established in concert with the enterprise-wide planning and budgeting process?
- Are capital budgeting decisions based upon demonstrated value to the institution after a comprehensive review of the priorities?
- Are needs assessed in the context of the institution's strategic imperatives and management objectives?

As complexity in healthcare and the IT industry increases, the role of the CIO has become much more strategic. In the past, it may have been acceptable for a CIO to be an "order taker," focusing on responsive solutions based on communicated expectations and requirements. During the past decade, however, the CIO has become a "facilitator," ensuring that users and technologies collaborated around the most effective use of technology to support the evolving needs of the institution. Moreover, the CIO is increasingly being called upon to be a leader and an "innovator," driving change and encouraging a more effective use of technology to support safety, security, savings and science.

In other words, **it has become critical for the CIO to be a partner with the CEO and other members of the executive team as this new role evolves.**

The CIO is also being called upon to demonstrate the value of the investments that have been made and are being made in emerging technologies. Healthcare organizations must scrutinize investments that are stressing and stretching the boundaries in ways that were previously unseen.

The CIO must effectively communicate the way information technologies can address this new challenge and assist the executive team through the priority setting processes that are now expected as part of the annual planning processes. The role of the CIO has also become one of providing justification for some IT investments. In the past a "sponsor" or a "champion" would be burdened with producing a cost-benefit analysis or a return-on-investment study. Now the CIO is frequently called upon to define the cultural and behavioral changes that must be realized to achieve the desired benefit from the introduction of new technologies.

PROJECT MANAGEMENT

Sam is also interested in assessing the project planning discipline and the technology development activities of his IT department. Although Sam appreciates that IT is not always an exact science, he wants to better understand the art that is associated with the deployment of new technologies. He also wants to better understand how well his IT staff members are serving as the custodians of scarce resources and how diligent they are in the world of uncertainty that often permeates new technology adoption and deployment.

Sam has developed the following list of questions to help with this assessment:

- How closely are project development timetables meeting the scheduled milestone dates?

- Are plans reliable and is planning being sufficiently inclusive?
- Is adequate testing and training incorporated into the plan?
- Are the actual development costs of IT projects exceeding the approved business plan projected developmental costs?
- With the increasing size and complexity of the investments in IT, what about cash flow projections?
- Can projections be relied on to manage my cash position? Are operating expenses of the various computer systems exceeding the projected operating expenses as stated in the originally proposed and approved business plans?
- Are proposed IT projects focusing on making hospital processes more efficient with quantifiable efficiency measures and will the articulated benefits actually be achieved?

Examples of solid project management assessment measures can include measuring the time it takes a physician in closing medical records for billing, turn around time for test results to be entered on to patients' records for discharge decisions, and other clinical processes that impact expense reduction and revenue improvement.

New and existing technology that may be of value for the hospital to consider purchasing or leasing should also be evaluated. Purchase decisions should include a value analysis, cost of implementation, operating and maintenance expenses, life cycle costs, the existing expenses, personnel and equipment that could be removed as a cost savings, and other projected efficiencies. If a return-on-investment can be demonstrated and the project was approved for implementation, what are the costs of missed project opportunities if the project implementation falls behind schedule?

IT should be focusing on how to obtain greater value from existing IT hardware and software. For example, some hospitals are finding that they already have the software capability of instituting bar code technology on patient wristbands, but the option was not activated when the system was initially installed because the bar code readers on patient units had not been purchased. Tremendous cost efficiencies can be obtained at low costs.

STAFF DEVELOPMENT

Sam is also concerned about staff development and succession planning. Because his CIO is investing a significant percentage of the available capital, Sam wants to be certain that the decisions being made are sustainable and that a change in leadership will not necessarily cause a change in direction for his IT strategies. Relevant questions include the following:

- Has the CIO been adequately attentive to education, training, and staff development?
- Is the staff sufficiently cohesive, while also being appropriately objective in the evaluation of alternative solutions?
- Are they considering best practices from around the country?
- Are they being constructively exposed to new industry literature, and thought leaders in healthcare and in IT?

PRODUCTIVITY AND COST MANAGEMENT

Obviously, one of Sam's concerns is also related to the total cost of ownership of his portfolio of IT solutions. He wants to understand his current investment as comprehensively as possible without getting into too much detail. He has identified some questions that he has asked his CIO to answer:

- Sam is convinced that his central IT department is attentive to costs, but are there hidden costs in the departments or divisions?
- Is there waste associated with distributed solutions that are not tightly integrated?
- Has the CIO been focused on simplification and the creation of a unifying platform that can be sustained?
- Are there reliable industry metrics that the CIO can use to compare his IT organization to others?
- With respect to forecasts, how far out can the future of IT be predicted?

Sam and his CIO are being presented with an opportunity to encourage the users to work collaboratively to define an architecture that can be sustained, well managed, and efficiently supported and enhanced. The creation of a cohesive culture focused on the most effective use of all capital resources to ensure business success and market differentiation should be the goal.

Sam's CIO can help Sam understand the right way to tackle this tough series of issues while demonstrating a commitment to quality and service excellence. The CIO can demonstrate that the cultural and behavioral changes needed to derive the greatest benefit are joint responsibilities and not solely in the hands of the CIO.

Varying business models are also surfacing in many boardrooms and executive sessions. Offshore programming services, application service providers and other hybrid solutions are gaining momentum in some corporate environments. Sam wants to be certain that he is aware of the possibilities and that his CIO is objectively evaluating the options.

ALTERNATE MANAGEMENT AND SUPPORT STRUCTURES

Sam has heard a great deal about outsourcing and wants to be certain he is educated about the possible alternatives. Sam wonders if there is a way to explore outsourcing without threatening the CIO and the IT staff. Is outsourcing or "hosting" a trend that should be considered?

Sam's CIO may be troubled by questions in this area. Industry trends seem to indicate that institutions are asking serious questions about outsourcing, or co-sourcing, and Sam needs to ask them as well. What is the total cost of my IT operation and how might costs be reduced? Do we really need to do all of the management internally? Over time, it is suggested that fewer CIOs will run their own networks and data centers, and more software development may be performed by others outside the enterprise. When this occurs, complexity sometimes increases, and Sam needs to be prepared to deal with the benefits and costs.

Sam is also seriously interested in the business skills of his CIO, particularly with regard to contract negotiations and vendor management (see the following sections). Sam wants to ensure that his CIO is aggressively negotiating with his suppliers and vendors. He should be using industry data and peer experiences to assist with the selection of systems development of vendor relationships, and the management of performance metrics. Sam is certain that good contracts lead to healthy relationships and strong partnerships.

Sam isn't certain, however, that his CIO has the skills needed to accomplish these goals. Sam will suggest that his CIO work more closely with colleagues in the institution in areas where negotiating and contracting skills are essential. This includes managed care contracting, facilities management, construction management, purchasing and materials management and financial management.

VENDOR MANAGEMENT, CONTRACT NEGOTIATIONS, AND CONTRACT MANAGEMENT

Sam can best support his CIO in this capacity by building a team, including the General Counsel, Purchasing Officer and CIO. By adding expertise to the process and by encouraging objectivity that will result from this teamwork, Sam and his CIO will be more successful.

FUTURE CONCERNS

Imagining the future is another component of Sam's role as the CEO. He needs to be prepared for a changing regulatory climate or unique reimbursement methodologies. He needs to understand the value of consumerism and the impact that it will have on his institution. Sam realizes that IT can play a role in addressing some of these issues.

Sam wants to know if his CIO and the IT staff are truly planning for the 'Digital Hospital of the Future.' He assembles another series of questions that revolve around how they can do a better job of predicting the future. In particular, he asks whether his management team is helping the CIO think differently about the challenges of the present in preparation for the challenges of the future? This is Sam's toughest, and perhaps most important, question.

As Dwight D. Eisenhower said, "The Plan is nothing, planning is everything." Sam knows that his CIO can add value by leading discussions about innovations and by driving business change. Sam no longer wants his CIO to be an order taker, or even a facilitator. Sam needs an innovator to drive business change.

Sam realizes that the above questions are not all-inclusive, but they can serve as a starting point to begin assessing the IT organization's performance. These and other routine assessment questions agreed upon by the CEO and CIO can help focus needed support and attention on optimizing return on the IT investment.

Terence T. Cunningham, III, MHA, FACHE, is the Hospital Administrator for Ben Taub General Hospital in Houston, a 650-bed academic medical center serving as the flagship teaching hospital for the Baylor College of Medicine. Ben Taub has been listed as one of the Top 100 Hospitals in the United States. Mr. Cunningham has worked with developing and managing information management activities as a senior healthcare executive for over 30 years. His assignments included the U.S. Air Force Medical Service at various hospitals and headquarters and Johns Hopkins Hospital. He has written and lectured extensively on total quality management and using continuous process improvement and continuous cost improvement in hospitals. Mr. Cunningham graduated with a BS in microbiology from California State University, Long Beach, and earned a masters degree in hospital administration from George Washington University in Washington, DC.

Stephanie L. Reel, MBA, is the Chief Information Officer and Vice Provost for Information Technology for the Johns Hopkins University, and Vice President for Information Services for Johns Hopkins Medicine. Ms. Reel earned a BS in information systems management from the University of Maryland and an MBA from Loyola College of Baltimore. The College of Healthcare Information Systems Executives named her CIO of the Year in 2000. Her innovations have been recognized by Computerworld and the Smithsonian Institute with an award that remains on display in the Smithsonian's Museum of American History. Ms. Reel is a member of the Board of Directors for the Microsoft Healthcare Users Group, the Healthcare Information Systems Executive Association, the GE Medical Systems Global Advisory Board, the College of Healthcare Information Systems Executives, HIMSS, the HealthCare Advisory Council, and the National Alliance for Health Information Technology. She also serves on the State of Maryland's Medical Privacy and Confidentiality Advisory Board.

References

1. Coile RC: *The Paperless Hospital: Healthcare in a Digital Age.* Chicago, IL: Health Administration Press/HIMSS; 2002: p 285.
2. *Implementation Guide for the Use of Bar Code Technology in Healthcare.* Chicago: HIMSS; 2003.

CHAPTER 6

The Grass Is Greener?
Outsourcing and the Merits of Marriage

Joseph E. Boyd, MBA

Unable to sleep, Sam Weatherspoon arrived at the office early this morning. He was still bothered by the concerns related to information technology that had occupied so much of his time yesterday. As he settled into his chair, he noticed yesterday's Wall Street Journal and reflected again on the outsourcing article he had read at lunch. Sam chuckled to himself as he considered the topic. Outsourcing. He couldn't think of a business concept that engendered more emotion!

Sam had noted through the years that leaders, particularly IT professionals, are completely polarized on this topic. Their reactions to the concept are visceral and sometimes almost irrational. Opponents of outsourcing seem to believe that the business practice carries with it a complete loss of control, a guaranteed mass layoff of staff, destruction of corporate culture and a guaranteed bad marriage to a gold digging spouse intent only on stealing their money and ideas. Proponents believe that outsourcing will allow them to take the most dysfunctional parts of their organizations, the ones that they least understand and care about, and turn them over to someone – anyone – who will deal with the problem and stem the hemorrhaging of money. Once the contract is signed they can forget about the problems that consume all of their time at work and rob them of valuable sleep at night.

Sam was also aware that both opponents and proponents of outsourcing could provide expert witnesses with powerful case studies and compelling arguments for or against the concept.

In fact, Sam knew that outsourcing is a business tool, pure and simple. As with any tool, it can be effective when applied correctly but a disaster if used improperly. He also suspected that it was not right for every organization or for every business function in a hospital.

"Well, there are no expert witnesses in my office at 5:30 in the morning," Sam thought. "Now is as good a time as any to formulate my own thoughts about what a balanced view of outsourcing, particularly IT outsourcing, should be."

He picked up a pad of paper and wrote, "Why do healthcare organizations look for outside IT partners?" He underlined the words twice, divided the page into "valid" and "invalid" columns and started to list the reasons.

After a half hour or so of thinking about the important reasons hospitals like Ingalls consider outsourcing, Sam pushed back from his desk and looked at his work. He concluded that there were three valid reasons, and two invalid ones, for doing so. In addition, there was another, more ambiguous category of reasons for outsourcing that were not so easily defined.

VALID REASONS FOR OUTSOURCING

Leveraging an Outsourcer's Capacity, Perspective and Expertise
The healthcare organization should take advantage of outsourcing. After all, IT is the business of these firms, not just a department within a healthcare delivery organization. It stands to reason that the organization should be able to have access to currency in general technology and specific healthcare applications by working with an outsourcer who has experience in a broad scope of industries and sufficient depth of experience in the healthcare IT world.

Minimizing the Fixed Cost Component of IT
If the organization needed temporary or infrequent expertise in a particular area, wouldn't it be smarter to have experts available on an as-needed basis rather than having to carry the cost of the expertise as a fixed component of the IT cost structure? A big technology firm should have people trained in almost any discipline that may be important to a healthcare organization now or down the road.

Leveraging the Outsourcer's Group Purchasing Power
If an IT outsourcer truly has leverage, it should be able to save the hospital money. Most organizations understand the savings it realizes from group purchasing agreements for supplies. The unit costs for running networks and computers, particularly if they can be consolidated into an outsourcing company's existing data centers and management systems, will almost certainly be lower than the hospital's costs if it made the purchases on its own.

INVALID REASONS FOR OUTSOURCING

Transferring a Problem Department or Component
A CEO can delegate tasks and responsibility but ultimately accountability must remain with the CEO and his or her team. One cannot eliminate one's problem by simply shoveling it away.

Commercializing an Internal IT Product
There are numerous examples of healthcare organizations deciding that they want to sell their internally-developed products and turn their IT organization into a profit center. These experiments did not work very well. First, hospitals and outsourcers are both generally service providers and are not particularly good at being in the product

business. Second, there was often a "Trojan horse" mentality on the part of other hospitals when it came to buying systems from competitors or potential competitors. Third, there should be a healthy skepticism about the efficacy of the joint marketing agreements or "writing a big check" for the asset arrangements. In the end, if the product was not a priority for the outsourcer, the sales did not seem to take off and the overall price of the outsourcing business suggested that the outsourcer made up for the "big check" in some other aspect of the outsourcing agreement. *(At the end of this item Sam had written and underlined the words, "If it sounds too good to be true, it probably is!")*

Ambiguous Reasons for Outsourcing

What was more interesting than the "valid" and "invalid" lists was a list of reasons that did not fit into either of these columns. These were indeed reasons for considering outsourcing but they were neither inherently valid nor invalid. This list included the following:

Allowing the Organization's CIO to Be More Strategic and Less Tactical

At Ingalls, for instance, the CIO is very smart and very aware of how technology can be used to improve relations with doctors and nurses and to give Ingalls a general competitive advantage. But the CIO always seemed to be busy with payroll issues, production cycle schedules, personnel performance reviews, or some other tactical part of IT. Could selective outsourcing allow the hospital to get more strategic use of his or her time?

Frustration with the Current IT Organization's Performance

Some healthcare organizations have been tempted to outsource their IT functions because the department seemed to be constantly in conflict with other hospital departments. Such reasoning is suspect. It is probable that organizations that do not first understand the reasons for a dysfunctional relationship between IT and the rest of the hospital are unlikely to eliminate the dysfunction through outsourcing.

Facing the Rigidity of a Contract

Having a confining contract with an outsourcing partner could mean that poorly estimated projects could cost "extra." The organization could get "nickled and dimed" if it did ensure that everything was spelled out in every task order and project plan. On the other hand, the threat of cost overruns should cause the hospital to become much more disciplined and rigorous when it comes to planning IT projects. If a department requests a project today and that project is not managed effectively, the cost overruns show up in the IT department budget and the "requesting" department does not bear direct financial responsibility. On the other hand, with outsourcing, the financial responsibility can be aligned with the department consuming the service. Perhaps managing an outsourcing partner, with constraints that are contractual and financial consequences that are visible, will cause the hospital to be more disciplined and hold IT more accountable.

While relatively brief, these lists capture some important things to consider when evaluating the outsourcing of IT.

SPECIFIC OBSERVATIONS ON
OUTSOURCING SELECTION CRITERIA

First, the valid reasons for considering outsourcing center on leverage and making structural changes in the cost of IT services. This does not always mean that current costs will improve dramatically. In many cases, it is wise to consider outsourcing alternatives if the decision can either: (1) shift the costs of IT from fixed to variable over time; or (2) reduce the amount of increase in IT spending over the long haul (e.g., instead of IT spending representing 5% of revenues as it does currently, it would represent 2.5% of revenues five years from now).

If an outsourcing arrangement does not have this type of financial characteristic, there is either something wrong with the relationship that is being negotiated or the outsourcing partner truly does not offer the organization sufficient leverage. In either case, the relationship does not make sense. What is important here is to focus on the leverage that can be enjoyed in the relationship, not the specific cost reductions. Leverage should lead to a favorable cost structure over the long haul. Excessive short-term focus on cost savings is likely to lead to a disappointing business relationship.

Second, the invalid reasons for outsourcing identified above were all related to attempts to transfer unsolved problems to a third party in hope that the problems would magically disappear. This is never a good reason to enter into an outsourcing relationship. The better an organization understands its costs and processes, the more successful it can be in negotiating the kind of relationship that really improves the hospital's performance.

Outsourcing relationships that are based on turning over a poorly understood business function will generally have one of two negative results: either (1) the outsourcing organization will make the process worse due to poor understanding of user needs, inadequate documentation, poorly aligned expectations, and the like; or (2) the outsourcer will discover how to optimize the process and provide the service for a fraction of the hospital's current cost, leading to accusations of price gouging and concerns over payments out of line with the benefits enjoyed by the hospital.

This does not mean that it is invalid to have some lesser understood processes included in an outsourcing arrangement. These dysfunctional elements, however, should not be the primary focus of the relationship. Cleaning up a few of these areas can be considered a latent benefit of outsourcing but it should not be the prime motivation.

Third, the most interesting category of reasons for outsourcing, the ambiguous one, raises questions regarding whether the hospital as a whole is prepared to make the cultural change and accept the additional rigor required to take on a partner. These cultural considerations are critical. A great deal of the analysis associated with why outsourcing arrangements succeed or fail focuses on factors such as communication, due diligence, proper expectations, appropriate service level negotiations, and governance. This focus is appropriate, and intelligently working through these factors is the key to a successful relationship.

An often-overlooked component in this research is the need to make an initial assessment of how culturally prepared a hospital is to take on a partner. Figure 6-1 contains a list of questions that may be instructive in assessing how culturally prepared a hospital might be to embrace IT outsourcing.

Possessing a corporate culture that is unaccustomed or even hostile toward "partnering" does not mean that outsourcing is impossible. It does mean that exceptional care will need to be taken in the structuring of the relationship and that contracting with an outsourcing consultant, which is always advisable, would be critical for the hospital.

- Does the corporate culture embrace change?
- Is the corporate culture more proactive than reactive?
- Do leaders set and subsequently measure departmental goals as a routine part of managing the effectiveness of departments within the hospital?
- Does the hospital have a rigorous performance management system?
- Do executives in the hospital have specific financial incentives to improve the economic performance for their areas of responsibility?
- Is the hospital comfortable with procuring services from and between hospital departments?
- Does the hospital have established transfer rates or some other measure for measuring services procured from other internal departments?
- Does the hospital avoid having redundant support services that are not shared between strategic business units?
- Does the hospital have formal standards of service for shared service departments such as human resources, financial services and IT?
- Has the hospital successfully joint ventured or partnered with other entities in core areas of its business?
- Are current IT initiatives evaluated based on improved economic performance of the hospital (ROI, ROA, payback period standards, and the like)?

The more "yes" answers, the greater the likelihood of success in an outsourcing relationship.

Figure 6-1. Assessing a Hospital's Overall Receptivity to Outsourcing

GENERAL OBSERVATIONS ON OUTSOURCING SELECTION CRITERIA

After evaluating the observations specifically related to the valid, invalid, and ambiguous reasons for outsourcing discussed above, several overarching ideas became clear to Sam Weatherspoon. First, to effectively outsource IT, his organization would need to be prepared to adopt a more disciplined approach to the way the hospital consumed IT resources. The hospital leadership would need to be sure that its CIO could be as effective managing a relationship as he or she had been at "getting things done." Having a third party accountable for the tactical aspects of IT execution should allow the hospital the luxury of having a strategically focused CIO role. Did they have the right person in the role?

Second, discipline and strategic focus would be necessary whether the organization decided to outsource some or all of the IT functions. After all, Ingalls would never consider outsourcing the strategic direction of IT for the hospital. Writing the lists had reinforced Sam's belief that the strategic planning for the hospital, which included the supporting IT strategy, should always remain an Ingalls' function. Therefore, a decision to do selective outsourcing versus total outsourcing of the execution of IT was simply a matter of deciding where the organization could get the most leverage with the least risk.

Finally, the process of writing the list had caused Sam to realize that it might be important to enforce service agreements between IT and the other departments now, with an internal IT organization, independent of whether they ever decided to make a move to outsource. The better all of the leadership team understood IT services needs and limitations, the more effective they could be at using IT effectively—whether outsourced or not.

SAM'S 21ST CENTURY IT DATING GUIDE FOR HOSPITALS

As Sam Weatherspoon thought more about outsourcing, he laughed as he realized how similar this business process is to a marriage. Some of the same concepts—diligence, trust and commitment—applied. There would need to be a courtship and romance, but both parties would also need to prepare for a longer, more familiar working partnership that characterizes most successful marriages. If they did it, they couldn't make this kind of commitment lightly! Could an old bachelor like Ingalls make the changes necessary to marry successfully? Sam wasn't sure. But the analogy was fun to think about at 6:00 in the morning. He poured himself another cup of coffee and decided to see how far he could extend the analogy.

Rule 1: Have a Clear Set of Objectives

Have a clear set of objectives for the relationship. Failed relationships can frequently be tracked back to poor communication and misaligned expectations of what marriage is all about. If an organization plans to enter into an outsourcing relationship, it must take responsibility for it and make sure it understands exactly what it wants. At the executive level, the hospital will need to have a clear, long-term but flexible plan for where it wants the relationship to go. This operational plan should be the foundation of the marriage contract.

Rule 2: Pick a Partner with the Right Culture and Capabilities

Pick a partner with the culture, style and capabilities best positioned to help realize that plan. This means that an organization must honestly assess its own strengths and weaknesses. Outsourcing firms are not all alike. A hospital must be particular in finding a partner that best complements the organization. A hospital must also ensure it has the processes and procedures in place to effectively manage the relationship and communicate appropriately between the two companies. A hospital and its outsourcing partner will need to function as one company in this area if the relationship is going to be successful.

Rule 3: Hire a Marriage Counselor

A matchmaker is needed because this is too important a decision for the organization's approach to be penny-wise and pound-foolish. There are a number of consulting firms that specialize in matchmaking in IT outsourcing. Before a hospital hires such a firm, though, it should have a clear vision for the outsourcing relationship and ensure that the consulting firm has creative ideas regarding how to guide the negotiation in a way that will meet the hospital's requirements. (A limited, non-exhaustive list of business outsourcing consulting firms is included at the end of this chapter.)

Rule 4: Marry for Love but Hire a Good Lawyer

In addition to needing a good marriage counselor, a good lawyer is necessary as well. There are a number of law firms that specialize in structuring complex long-term contracts. It is a very good idea to use such a firm during contracting. As with hiring the marriage counselor/business consultant, before a hospital hires a legal consultant, it should explain the organization's long term plan for the outsourcing relationship and ensure the law firm has creative ideas regarding how to structure a contract to meet the hospital's needs. (A limited, non-exhaustive list of law firms that provide this service is included at the end of this chapter.)

Rule 5: The Counselor and the Lawyer Will Leave after the Reception

Both the marriage counselor and the lawyer will go home after the reception. The senior hospital representative, preferably the CIO, who will be responsible for managing the outsourcing relationship, must drive the negotiations. The outsourcing consultant and outside counsel should support the negotiation but never lead it.

Rule 6: Raise the Veil Before You Kiss

The outsourcer's account executive who will be responsible for meeting the hospital's IT needs should be active in the negotiations. That person must be someone whom the hospital respects and trusts. That person must have authority to make the relationship work. If the outsourcing organization cannot or will not assign that person to the account in advance of completing the negotiation, the wedding should be called off.

Rule 7: Listen to the Voices of Experience

Listen to others who have experience with these marriages. A hospital should talk to other organizations that have entered into outsourcing relationships and visit with them if possible. An organization should gather as much knowledge as it can prior to making a commitment.

Rule 8: Be Prepared to Make Some Changes

Old bachelors can get set in their ways. An outsourcing partner will force an organization to change some of the ways it acquires IT services, measures results, and interacts between departments. An organization must prepare itself for the change. It must set reasonable expectations and make a concerted effort to make the relationship work.

Further Thoughts on the Rules

Sam's analogy, while not perfect, covers a great deal of important territory. Most of the items are self-explanatory but a few merit some further discussion. For example, Rule 2 related to cultural fit is important when the outsourcing entity is local. It is absolutely critical when a relationship with an offshore outsourcer is contemplated. The normal challenges associated with managing an outsourcing relationship are amplified when trying to coordinate with a partner that is off site.

In an interview with Thomas Claburn, Forrester research analyst John McCarthy suggests that successful management of offshore resources requires particular attention to governance:[1]

- How well aligned are business and IT?
- Are they at each other's throats all the time?
- How sophisticated are your IT processes?
- How rigorous are they?
- Are you used to things like service-level agreements?

These all dictate how easy or relatively easy it will be to manage the offshore provider.

These governance issues are important in any outsourcing relationship but they are critical when an organization is working with people thousands of miles away. McCarthy also warns in the same article that offshore outsourcing is still a bit of a fad and that the general ramp-up to a meaningful investment in offshore outsourcing will take a long time to accomplish.

There is no doubt that some readers of Rules 3 and 4 above will argue that it is unnecessary to hire either an outsourcing consultant or outside legal counsel with experience in outsourcing, much less both. This is not the situation in which to be frugal. If an organization is doing a full scale outsourcing of IT, the investment it makes in these services during the selection and due diligence processes alone will pay for itself multiple times during the full term of a typical five-to-ten year relationship.

These consultants will also help an organization understand market standards in the terms that are negotiated, minimize both financial and business risks, and instill a structure and discipline in the processes associated with acquiring outsourcing services. These consultants can also provide valuable assistance when it comes to approaching organized labor discussions that can be affected by outsourcing arrangements. They can also help to develop a plan to communicate effectively with affected communities outside the hospital, such as local government agencies, physicians' groups, and the local press.

Any time a large employer makes labor force changes, it is wise to seek the advice of experts who can help with planning and communication. As Sam points out in Rule 6, the responsibility for the relationship and the contract still rests with the hospital. The selection process should be led by the hospital, but good managerial and legal consulting assistance is a very wise investment.

Rule 7, "Listen to the voices of experience," is probably the most important rule on Sam's list. However, it is astonishing how frequently this common sense advice is ignored. Prior to making a decision to explore outsourcing, it is imperative that the executives responsible for making the decision talk to other executives in companies with outsourcing experience. This reference checking should not be limited to the CIO. The outsourcing of such an important service area impacts most, if not all, departments in a hospital. As much of the hospital leadership as is financially possible should actively interview comparable contacts in hospitals where IT has been outsourced.

Conducting this type of broad-based interview provides a number of benefits. First, it allows an organization to take advantage of the experience of others. Second, it helps to signal to the organization itself that change is about to occur. Third, it provides departmental leadership with a sense of the adjustments that will be necessary in order to make a relationship work. It is not sufficient to merely check with references provided by prospective outsourcing partners, nor should visits be limited to people and institutions that are like-minded. The broader the experience an organization can garner through this process, the better prepared it will be to have a successful outsourcing relationship.

SINGLE VERSUS MARRIED LIFE

Sam decided, in fairness, that he should probably consider the reasons why Ingalls may want to consider staying single. He flipped a page in his note pad and started his third list of the day.

First, if, after dating a bit, we determine that there really isn't a partner out there who can get us where we want to go faster or less expensively, there is no compelling reason to make a change.

Second, if we come to the conclusion that the culture of the hospital simply is not compatible with the style of any IT outsourcing organization that we can find, this type of marriage should never be risked.

Third, simply using "loss of control" as a reason for not considering outsourcing does not make good business sense. However, a lack of sufficient controls to manage a partner can be a good reason. It would be unwise to enter into such a relationship if Ingalls does not have the internal controls and properly positioned executives to manage it. If Ingalls is not yet ready to manage such an important relationship, we should not consider marriage.

Once again, Sam's relatively short list contains some important information. If an organization does not believe that it can obtain leverage from an outsourced IT department, there is no real reason to do it. Leverage, much more than cost savings, should be the primary driver. If an IT department can be just as efficient independently, it is sufficient to simply benchmark IT costs periodically to ensure they continue to be efficient and competitive.

Second, if an organization lacks the processes and controls to manage a third party relationship, then improving those processes, not outsourcing, should be the top priority of an IT organization. Focus on process improvement in this area will improve both the quality and efficiency of the IT department over the relative short run. A well managed IT department should be capable of selectively outsourcing some or all functions at any given time if market conditions warrant that decision.

Third, corporate culture is important. It is sometimes referred to as the gyroscope of an organization in that it is highly resistant to movement in any direction. If an organization's corporate culture does not favor partnerships, an outsourcing relationship is not likely to be successful. If the hospital culture is resistant to outsourcing, and outsourcing is still being considered, it would be wise to make some interim moves that serve to move the culture closer to one where outsourcing can be successful. Any "no" answers that were provided to the questions in Figure 6-1, on page 91, will provide a good indication of some interim areas in which to begin that work.

SUMMARY

Sam looked up from his desk and noticed that his administrative assistant was trying to signal that his 8:30 a.m. appointment had arrived 10 minutes early and was anxious to see him. He signaled that he understood and asked her to give him a minute. He wanted a few seconds to draw some conclusions from his morning's work.

While Sam's marriage analogy had not held up completely, it had helped him sort out his thinking in this area. He knew that until and unless Ingalls was properly prepared, it should not consider nuptials. He also thought that it would be healthy to explore a bit of dating even if the hospital was not yet ready for marriage. Sam was convinced that it was foolish to start a serious relationship without first seeking the advice of colleagues and professional organizations that could help guide his organization in the right direction. Finally, and most importantly, Ingalls should have a clear plan for how IT could support the hospital's overall strategy. Ingalls should only consider an IT partnership if that move could help the hospital achieve its objectives faster and less expensively than it could on its own.

Sam closed his notepad and signaled his assistant that he was ready to face the beginning of another day.

Joseph E. Boyd, MBA, has over 20 years of information technology experience with Electronic Data Systems, KPMG Peat Marwick, GTE and Perot Systems. At Perot Systems, Mr. Boyd held a variety of positions from 1990 to 1994, when he was named Vice President and General Manager for the Healthcare Industry practice. In 1997, Mr. Boyd was promoted to Executive Vice President and General Manager for Perot Systems North American operations, directing over 4,000 employees in a $600M business that included seven industry verticals. Mr. Boyd retired from Perot Systems in 2001 but continues to be involved in the industry, providing management consulting services through his own firm, Boyd Consulting. Mr. Boyd also serves as the Chairman of Healthlink Incorporated. He holds a BA in history and an MBA from Mississippi State University.

References

1. Claburn T: Report: Offshore Outsourcing Often Still More the Exception than the Rule. *Information Week.* Dec 15, 2003; Article ID: 16700603.

Bibliography

Cohen LR, Scardino L, Stone L: Predictions for Outsourcing in 2004. Gartner Research. Dec 11, 2003; Note Number: SPA-21-4390.

Gabler J: Predictions for Healthcare Management Strategies in 2004. Gartner Research. Dec 16, 2003; Note Number: SPA-21-6595.

Goolsby K: Taking Pains with a Hospital's Transition to Outsourcing. Outsourcing Center: An Everest Group Company. Available at www.outsourcing-healthcare.com.

Overview of Outsourcing Transactions That Work. TPI Publications. Available at www.tpi.net/pdf/overview of outsourcing transactions that work.pdf.

APPENDIX A
OUTSOURCING BUSINESS AND LEGAL CONSULTING

These lists are arranged alphabetically. They are in no way meant to be exhaustive. Information provided about these firms was taken directly from the firms' respective Web sites. The information was either summarized or modified for readability only. Organizations that offer both outsourcing consulting and outsourcing services were excluded from this list. Inclusion in this list does not imply endorsement.

Business Outsourcing Consultants

Clearwater Management Consultants

8111 LBJ Freeway, Suite 1150, Dallas, TX 75251
PH: 214-219-2815
www.clearviewmgmnt.com

Clearwater Management Consultants, LLC (CMC) has a practice area specifically focused on achievement of quality improvement through a collaborative development of client-specific service level management programs. Their services include assistance with definition, prioritization, measurement and monitoring of specific performance levels for the organization.

The Everest Group

12700 Preston Road, Suite #190, Dallas, TX 75230
PH: 972-980-0013
www.everestgrp.com

The Everest Group is one of the world's most prominent consulting organizations assisting corporations and governments in procuring and managing outsourcing relationships. It teaches buyers how to manage outsourcing relationships and can help an organization do the following: identify and define what processes to outsource; transition work to the supplier (internal or external); get more from a relationship; renegotiate a contract; arrange early termination; extend a relationship; test the market; or bring services back in-house.

TPI

10055 Grogan's Mill Road, Suite 200, The Woodlands, TX 77380
PH: 281-465-5700
www.tpi.net

TPI has advised on over 550 sourcing transactions with a total contract value of more than $330 billion since its inception in 1989. Its primary focus is to assist clients with the evaluation, negotiation, implementation and management of IT and business process sourcing initiatives. Employing more than 150 advisors who average more than 21 years of industry experience, TPI assists corporations throughout the Americas, Europe and Asia Pacific. Its mission is "To help clients make informed, lasting and substantial improvements in their performance through the use of sourcing."

Legal Outsourcing Consultants

Baker & McKenzie

International Executive Offices, One Prudential Plaza, 130 E. Randolph Drive, Suite 2500, Chicago, IL 60601

PH: 312-861-8800

www.bakerinfo.com

Baker & McKenzie's IT practitioners have the requisite skills to handle any type of technology deal. Their attorneys are well-versed in both the legal and technical aspects of technology transfers, service level agreements, equipment design, fulfillment, application agreements, and e-commerce arrangements.

Milbank, Tweed, Hadley & McCloy LLP

1 Chase Manhattan Plaza, New York, NY 10005-1413

PH: 212-530-5000

www.milbank.com

Milbank's information technology lawyers, located throughout the firm's global network of offices, have a wide array of experience with computers, software, outsourcing, Internet, e-commerce, and new media, and are on the leading edge of business trends in the high technology sector.

CHAPTER 7

The CEO–CIO Relationship: A Roundtable Discussion

Moderator
Detlev H. (Herb) Smaltz, PhD, FHIMSS, CHE, CKM: Associate Professor in Health Informatics and Chief Technology Officer, UAB Health System

Participants
Russell P. Branzell, CHE, FHIMSS: CIO, Poudre Valley Health System
David Hoidal, MHA: CEO, UAB Health System
Michael W. Murphy, CPA: CEO, Sharp HealthCare
William A. Spooner: CIO, Sharp HealthCare
Rulon F. Stacey, PhD: CEO, Poudre Valley Health System
Michael R. Waldrum, MD, MS: CIO, UAB Health System

Much has been written over the last decade or so about the role of the CIO. In many organizations, particularly those in highly competitive markets, the role of the IT department has evolved from a back-room support function to a strategic driver with the potential to transform an organization. Increasingly, CIOs have become formal members of their respective organizations' senior management team, and many now report directly to the CEO. However, the popular press suggests that many CIOs have not yet acclimated to the very different environment of senior executives. Articles such as *The Mars/Pluto Relationship,*[1] *Chasm Closer: The CIO/CEO Gap Still Dogs IS,*"[2] and *Hatred: An Update (CIO-CEO Relationships)*[3] are but a few sample titles that suggest that CIOs need to do a better job building relationships with their senior executive peers, and particularly with the CEO.

This chapter takes the form of a roundtable discussion to explore the relationship between CEOs and CIOs from the perspective of three highly effective healthcare organizations. The first is Sharp Healthcare, the largest health system and the largest private-sector employer in San Diego, with four acute care hospitals, four specialty hospitals, three medical groups, and a health plan. Representing Sharp HealthCare are CEO Mike Murphy and CIO Bill Spooner. The second is Poudre Valley Health System, a five-hospital system based in Fort Collins, Colorado. The organization is represented by CEO Rulon Stacey and CIO Russ Branzell. The third organization is the University of Alabama at Birmingham (UAB) Health System, a multi-hospital academic medical center. Representing UAB Health System are CEO David Hoidal and CIO Mike Waldrum. All three CIO participants in this roundtable discussion report directly to their respective CEOs. Biographies for all participants can be found at the end of this chapter.

CRITICAL FACTORS IN THE CEO/CIO RELATIONSHIP

[Herb Smaltz] **The subject of this chapter is the relationship between the CEO and CIO. Can you each describe the nature of the relationship you have with one another and what you see as the critical success factors for an effective professional relationship between a CEO and a CIO? Let's start first with the CEOs and then finish up with the CIOs.**

[Michael Murphy] The CIO of our organization reports directly to me and serves as a critical member of our organization's senior management team. We have a very open and professional relationship and he provides the organization and me with leadership in the areas of IT and communications. He plays an active role in our discussions and decision regarding strategic direction and resource allocation for the entire enterprise. The most critical success factors for our effective relationship are communication, respect and leadership. We must also recognize and appreciate the needs of the entire organization and be able to think outside of our individual area of leadership.

[Rulon Stacey] My relationship with the CIO in our system is excellent on both a personal and a professional level. I have great personal respect for him and I believe that is important as we put together our future strategies. With that foundation, on a professional level I feel like my main job is to simply not interfere with what he is doing. I believe that he is the CEO of our Information Systems division, and as such, I believe it is important to stay out of his way and let him get the things done that he thinks are important. He is an integral part of our senior management team and is completely a part of the strategies that we set as a system. However, when those strategies are set, I expect that he is fully capable of creating an IT strategy that will support our overall direction. I am fortunate enough to work with a CIO who generates this amount of trust. If he were not as capable as he is, I believe that it would hinder our ability to function this way.

[David Hoidal] My relationship with the CIO is a very close and collaborative one. We discuss and evaluate all major decisions and initiatives and we often discuss strategy and alignment of stakeholders especially as it relates to IT. We, in fact, support each other in this regard.

An effective relationship with the CIO requires the CEO's willingness to remain up to speed on all the hot IT topics in the marketplace. The CEO must at all times have an open mind when considering information systems but must be able to look beyond even several years to understand how everything will eventually tie together. As with any truly effective relationship, no punches should be pulled. The CEO and CIO must be able to communicate openly and honestly. After decisions are made, the CEO must be a proponent of the technology while at the same time, the CIO needs to ultimately follow the CEO's strategic agenda even when it may conflict periodically with a particular IT direction the CIO may want to explore.

[William Spooner] We have a collaborative, supportive relationship. Critical success factors involve the CEO and executive team committing the necessary time and effort to help construct an effective IT strategy and governance. All of senior leadership must be able to articulate and publicly support the IT strategy and goals, as we all must with regard to all our strategic objectives.

[Russell Branzel] Our relationship is open, collaborative, positively challenging and innovative. We have honest communication without any hidden agendas. A team environment where all win together is the basis of effective CEO/senior executive team relationships.

[Michael Waldrum] I report directly to the CEO; however I don't let this reporting relationship influence our working relationship. We have a very honest and frank relationship. Nothing is out of bounds for discussion. This open communication that flows in both directions is vital. He understands that the decisions that I am making are for the benefit of the enterprise and the patients we treat. Having mutual trust and aligned objectives is essential to managing in our complex enterprise. This open and collaborative problem resolution methodology extends to all members of the executive team. We have created a management forum for the executive team that is a safe harbor for discussion. In this forum the executives can discuss and deliberate any issue without fear. It is designed to discuss issues and problems and plans for resolution. It is not a forum to show all the great things that are being done.

MEASUREMENT OF THE CIO

[Herb Smaltz] **For the CEOs, what are your expectations of the CIO and how do you and/or your board of directors measure the CIO and his/her organization against those expectations?**

[Michael Murphy] My expectations of the CIO are to provide leadership of our senior management team in establishing the strategic direction and priorities of the endless IT needs and to play an active role with the team in establishing the strategic direction and priorities for the overall system. He plays an active role in working with the various stakeholders to ensure that their issues and concerns are factored in to the overall direction of the organization. He provides the leadership to assemble a skilled and motivated IT team that works well with the many stakeholders and successfully implements the IT services that we undertake. Our board of directors has an IT committee that works closely with the CIO and the senior leadership team in strategic direction and approval and review of significant IT capital projects. Success is measured based on various financial targets, service targets, user satisfaction targets, and delivering on the value proposition for the IT tools that we prioritize.

[Rulon Stacey] I expect that the CIO will fulfill the IT portion of our vision statement. We are in business to provide world class healthcare. To fulfill this vision, we have established six strategic objectives that every person in the organization needs

to support. The CIO has worked with his team to create a strategy in support of our strategic objectives, and they have listed their goals and how well they achieve them on a monthly basis in their own balanced score card. So, it is very easy to know what is expected of the CIO and the entire IT team because I can quickly glance at their balanced score card. However, I also expect that our CIO will be a part of the larger community in our organization and in the nation. I believe that it is important for the CIO to participate in our health system in areas other than just IT. To his credit, he is a vital player in our quality improvement process, joint venture boards of directors, and other areas. He is also involved on a national level with his professional organizations, which I think is critical in order to ensure that we are staying on top of the latest developments.

[David Hoidal] I expect the CIO to apply the organization's strategic initiatives as well as mission statement to the evaluation of IT needs. Most of the modern CIO's job is consumed with needs to integrate many disparate medical information systems and evaluate software in support of the electronic medical record. Aside from the bells and whistles, the CIO must evaluate the financial, strategic, and cultural impact that any changes might have both internally and externally. Because highly skilled healthcare IT personnel are extremely valuable and not abundant in the marketplace, the CIO must be able to allocate human capital as judiciously as financial capital.

Just as important is the ability to effectively align key stakeholders before, during, and after the purchase and to be an effective project champion or manager throughout the implementation phase.

WHAT DO CIOS NEED FROM CEOS?

[Herb Smaltz] **For the CIOs, what do you need from your CEO in order to be successful?**

[William Spooner] I need his public and private support. I need IT resource needs to be considered on an equal basis with all budgetary concerns—both operating and capital.

[Russell Branzell] This is what I need: clear strategic objectives with appropriate support and resources; prioritized projects; and direct feedback and guidelines on areas of improvement.

[Michael Waldrum] I need trust, confidence, and authority in addition to acceptance of failure. I also need him to understand that "failures" usually can't be attributed to one individual (i.e., the CIO) and that implementations require engagement and active problem solving from the business units as well as IT.

IDEAL ATTRIBUTES FOR AN EFFECTIVE CIO:
THE CEO'S PERSPECTIVE

[Herb Smaltz] **From the CEO's perspective, what attributes (i.e., specific skills and/or background) are ideal in order to be an effective CIO in today's healthcare environment and why?**

[Michael Murphy] The CIO must be a good team player—a good communicator, someone who is well versed in the IT field but who recognizes the clinicians' and patients' concerns and needs. Someone who understands the overall healthcare industry challenge and is able to inspire the confidence not only of the technology team but of the many other stakeholders who rely on the CIO and his or her team for their tools.

[Rulon Stacey] Leadership. I don't believe that it is enough to simply be knowledgeable in IT to be an effective CIO. Rather, I think it is critical for someone to be capable to be the CEO of his or her respective area. I actually think that it is more important to be a good leader than it is to be a good IT person. It is more important to create the strategy for the organization and to be effective in implementing that strategy than it is to know the nuts and bolts of the IT world. If someone is capable of being an effective leader, then I think that the other parts of being an effective CIO will fall into place.

[David Hoidal] Being a practicing physician, especially in an academic medical center, has been very helpful to me. We are fortunate to have such a person with us right now. However, this is not a criterion as long as the CIO understands the concept of a service orientation towards physicians. I think it almost goes without saying that broad-based experience as well as a passion for IT are essential. The ability to determine and understand the current state, to be a project champion, and to put the right people in the right places are all ideal as well.

PROCESS FOR EVALUATING NEW IT PROJECTS AND DETERMINING BUDGETS

[Herb Smaltz] **What is your organization's process for evaluating new IT projects and for determining how much money (operational and capital) is spent each year on IT?**

[Michael Murphy] Our organization's IT capital needs are evaluated along the same lines as all our capital projects. First priorities are given to business projects (e.g., obsolete CT scanner or telephone switch) and patient safety and patient quality investments, whether they are IT or clinical or plant maintenance. The remaining capital is allocated to individual projects based on expressed business cases from our various stakeholders that will drive the organization toward achieving our strategic directions. In reality there are far more projects then there is capital, so our senior management team spends considerable time prioritizing our limited resources. In IT and in all other aspects of capital allocation, it is incumbent on the senior leaders to educate our team on the need for the project and select those that allow us to best achieve our goals.

[Rulon Stacey] To be honest, our process needs improvement. In the past we have not had as much direction in this area as we have needed. This has left the organization to go in many different directions and caused our IT department huge problems in trying to keep so many people with so many different systems happy. One of the reasons why I feel that leadership is important is because an effective CIO, such as the one I work with now, is able to address this issue across many different department lines. This happens by explaining the problem, presenting a solution, and then generating support for the future process. That is what has happened in our organization as the CIO met

with the rest of the senior management group and presented the entire problem. He has developed a tool to analyze different projects and effectively solicited the support of the rest of senior management to implement the change. This is the value of an effective leader in this position.

[David Hoidal] At the heart of our organization is a highly competitive and cutting-edge medical school ranked in the top 20 in NIH funding. Naturally, we are very decentralized in our approach to new initiatives. Almost anyone can come up with an idea and it will get evaluated. After that, we do have the formal processes in place for prioritizing and bringing things up to the board. If the return on investment is there and it has broad-based appeal, we will find a way to get it funded.

[William Spooner] We have an annual process in which we update our five-year financial plan. The objective is to assure ourselves from a financial perspective that we can support our bond rating. It involves creation of pro forma income statement and cash flow projections. The cash flow projection determines the dollar amount of available capital. All entities submit capital proposals with supporting justification, which we evaluate based on contribution to our financial, service and quality goals. We conduct a collaborative exercise among senior leadership to perform the evaluation and negotiate the final capital spending priorities.

Operating budgets are similarly projected in conjunction with the capital planning effort. We calculate target expenses based on historical spending and planned changes. Final operating numbers are negotiated as we work to achieve an overall profitability target to support the cash flow and capital plan.

[Russell Branzell] The operational budget is determined based upon zero-based analysis plus ups/downs based on organizational needs. The capital budget is strategic objectives-based with prioritization determined by the informatics committee and senior management.

[Michael Waldrum] We have operational budget processes and capital budget processes that occur each year. There is no set amount carved out for IT. The entities have separate processes and we are involved in both. Coordination occurs by being involved in both and by participants in the IS executive committee.

MOST SIGNIFICANT IT CHALLENGES

[Herb Smaltz] **I'd like to put some organizational context on the discussions we've been having so far. What do each of you see as the most significant IT challenges faced by your organization?**

[Michael Murphy] There are many significant IT challenges that healthcare organizations face. These include limited capital, products that do not scale to the size of organization, products that are not really ready for prime time, lack of standardization within the health system that compromises the products' success, people's reluctance to change which underutilizes some products' ability to enhance processes, and the significant difficulty in interfacing the various products that various stakeholders believe they must have.

[Rulon Stacey] Access to capital. We have so many changes facing us as we grow that it is getting harder and harder to get the capital we need to be successful. The problem is that in order to make IT successful, it seems to take such a disproportionate amount of the capital that it generates an amount of frustration with the rest of the organization. I don't know that there is a way out of this. I don't expect IT prices to decrease, and I don't see our dependency on IT solutions decreasing.

[David Hoidal] There are so many different types of systems and no single solution. Accurate billing, electronic medical records, provider order entry, and clinical trial management are only a few of the ones we are faced with here. No one vendor has been able to address all of these issues and much of the needed functionality today cuts across multiple systems. So the healthcare system, rather than the industry, is left to bear the cost and the burden of making everything work together. And with resources the way they are in this age, it is always a challenge.

[William Spooner] Maintaining a robust infrastructure under severe budget constraints; effectively evaluating, prioritizing and funding proposed IT initiatives in a loosely confederated organization; continuing to challenge and motivate a seasoned, long-tenured management team and maintaining a high level of customer service consistently over time.

[Russell Branzell] Far greater demand for services than supply can meet. This forces prioritization and strategic focus.

[Michael Waldrum] The most significant IT challenge we face is enterprise integration of technology, information and processes. Our organization, like many academic medical centers, has a complex governance and organizational structure. This structure was not built to maximize problem resolution when it comes to IT or information management problems. Solving these problems across the organization is a significant challenge. In support of enterprise integration acceptance of certain standards is essential; however, this poses significant challenges for us.

IT'S SUCCESSES IN THE HEALTHCARE INDUSTRY

[Herb Smaltz] **Broadening the context a bit more, where has IT been a clear success in the healthcare industry?**

[Michael Murphy] There are countless areas of IT success in our organization and all of healthcare. Where would our industry be and how would we function without our ERP systems, patient registration, billing, clinical data repositories, the technology imbedded in so many clinical tools, transcription. Name a function that is performed in healthcare and IT is involved in its success.

[Rulon Stacey] Patient safety is, I believe, the biggest success. There is no doubt that patients in the U.S. are safer today than they were just a few years ago, largely because of the IT successes that have taken the variability of human error out of the equation in many areas. The IT revolution in medical records, bar coding, provider order entry and other areas have been dramatic, and it seems to me that they show no signs of stopping.

However, as I mentioned above, each new system and each new solution seems to be getting more expensive.

[David Hoidal] IT has been a clear success, especially as it relates to patient safety. Clearly, provider order entry has decreased medical errors tremendously. Automated drug dispensing systems and automated infusion pumps have great potential. I believe this is the area where IT will continue to make great strides. Being able to use computer logic in order to build in warnings, appropriate drug ranges, or drug interactions for clinical staff when they might otherwise be distracted, tired, or spread too thin is a tremendous opportunity that I hope we take full advantage of.

[William Spooner] IT has been a clear success in automating repetitive tasks whether financial or clinical. It has shown success in enabling patient safety, supply chain and revenue cycle improvements.

[Russell Branzell] Inpatient financial, business and clinical systems have been clear successes.

[Michael Waldrum] Access to clinical information; decreased process time for medication administration with provider order entry, and some limited decision support. There are a number of clear successes with patient management and accounting systems.

IT'S DISAPPOINTMENTS IN THE HEALTHCARE INDUSTRY

[Herb Smaltz] **Conversely, where does IT continue to be a disappointment in the industry?**

[Michael Murphy] The disappointment to me has been that while the advances are many, they are usually accomplished in silos or single purpose products that then must be cobbled together. Interfacing of these products is costly and often times of limited benefit. There are not enterprise solutions that deliver desired functionality to even the majority of the users, much less all of the users. I have also been disappointed that many of the products are not really ready for prime time when they are sold. Yet I remind myself of what I said above: where would we be without the advances we have made?

[Rulon Stacey] I believe that there is opportunity to improve in the area of a true electronic medical record. While we have made great strides, I hope that someday we could really get to a point where we could have a paperless system. Right now when people talk of going paperless, they really mean "reduced" paper work. I would like to see if there truly is an option to go paperless. I would also argue that there is an opportunity for improvement in the area of voice recognition. I make these suggestions again, knowing that the possibility of paying for all these new tools is going to be diminishing.

[David Hoidal] As I noted earlier, it's disappointing that the lack of functionality that cuts across multiple applications leaves healthcare systems like ours to bear the cost and the burden of making everything work together. Beyond issues relating to integrated functionality, I think that IT is not necessarily a disappointment in the sense that it is us, the people who run health systems (and by that, I mean the doctors, nurses,

administrators, third parties and the government) who dictate what IT should and should not become. When you think about the potential advantages related to having a nationally accessible, longitudinal patient record for example, it is disappointing to think that because of our fragmented system, it will be such a formidable task. Who would own it, who would run it and how would power shift among payors and providers as a result of such a decision?

[William Spooner] Systems don't always support productive workflows effectively. At the same time, IT professionals have not been consistently effective with their companies in process improvement necessary to gain full advantage of their IT systems. IT vendors have fared poorly in creating interoperable systems. Vendors and customers alike have been ineffective in standardizing database elements, processes, and the like that would support interoperability.

[Russell Branzell] Integration of the entire community of care, which includes inpatient, outpatient and emergency departments, plus private physician offices.

[Michael Waldrum] Vendor solutions and vendor productivity continue to disappoint users and organizations. Adoption of technology and use of technology in healthcare delivery organizations has been slow. There is a lack of unified standards and interoperability within and among healthcare delivery organizations. The potential for use of information to improve healthcare delivery within organizations and improve healthcare delivery across the country has been disappointing. There is enormous potential for IT to improve healthcare delivery and there are many impediments to adoption of IT. Healthcare organizations and the providers who operate within these organizations need incentives and resources to realize the great potential that IT has to offer. Hopefully the national healthcare information infrastructure movement to enhance the interoperability issues, combined with the creation of an incentive system, will lead to acceleration of IT adoption within healthcare organizations.

SUMMARY

[Herb Smaltz] I'll attempt to sum up the common themes that were expressed in this discussion along with some elaboration. We started our discussion at an individual relationship level and expanded the scope and context to include organizational and industry effects, since relationships are forged within specific contexts.

Clearly, a disappointing lack of standardization and integration between and among vendors' healthcare applications coupled with tight capital budgets creates a difficult context within which CIOs operate. On the bright side, the federal spotlight and healthcare application accreditation/certification processes[4] are beginning to put greater pressure on vendors to create products that truly, at the least, interoperate. Beyond applications and funding issues, CIOs must also operate in highly complex organizational structures with multiple, sometimes opposing, stakeholder groups.

As the CEOs in this roundtable noted, such an environment requires leadership attributes first and foremost in the person of the CIO. In fact, I would venture to suggest that based on a large literature base, validated by the responses of the CEOs in this roundtable, the first fundamental characteristic of solid CEO-CIO relationships is the presence of leadership qualities in both individuals. Beyond leadership attributes, additional basic principles for building and sustaining excellent CEO-CIO relationships include:

- Honest and open communications (no subject out of bounds; discussion without attribution);
- Collaboration;
- Being able to think and contribute outside of one's individual functional area of leadership;
- Clearly articulated governance and decision rights (ambiguity in this area can damage relationships and effectiveness);
- Measuring performance (perception often kills relationships and credibility; measure every aspect of IT service deliver; data is the only trump card that is useful against perception); and
- Aligning IT strategy with business strategy such that it's simply "strategy."

The most important observation that one should take away from this chapter is that interpersonal attributes and/or interactions are only part of the CEO-CIO relationship formula. They are a necessary, but not sufficient, component of an excellent CEO-CIO relationship. Equally important are some organizational structures (e.g., IT governance structure and decision rights) and processes (e.g., measuring IT service delivery) that create openness and transparency about how IT-related decisions are made and that constantly show the value added by IT and the services delivered by the CIO and the rest of the IT department.

These final organizational components of the formula create enduring professional credibility and trust, which are the other important fundamentals of solid CEO-CIO relationships.

Russell P. Branzell, CHE, FHIMSS, is the Chief Information Officer and Vice President of Information Services for Poudre Valley Health System in Fort Collins, Colorado, a "Most Wired"/"Most Wireless" health system. Under Mr. Branzell's leadership, Poudre Valley also earned Information Week's *Top 500 Award for innovative technology usage and also received the Business Technology Optimization Excellence Award for IT Governance Best Practices. Prior to joining Poudre Valley, Mr. Branzell served in numerous leadership positions at Sisters of Mercy Health System based in St. Louis, Missouri, where his positions included Regional Deputy CIO, Corporate Executive Director and various director-level assignments. He also held numerous CIO positions during his 13 years in the U.S. Air Force. He is a Fellow in HIMSS and a board certified Diplomate in the American College of Healthcare Executives.*

David Hoidal, MHA, is CEO of UAB Health System, where he previously served as Chief Operating Officer, overseeing the daily operations of the University Hospital, the Callahan Eye Foundation Hospital and The Kirklin Clinic. Prior to coming to UAB, Mr. Hoidal was the Senior Vice President and Chief Operating Officer of Tulane University Hospital and Clinics in Louisiana. Prior to joining Tulane, he served as CEO of DePaul/Tulane Behavioral Health Center in New Orleans as well as CEO for HCA Peninsula Hospital in Hampton, Virginia. Mr. Hoidal has received the HCA award for Outstanding Operations, has acted as an HCA Quality Assurance Surveyor, and has been named one of Healthweek's Top 25

Turnaround CEOs. He received his BA in psychology from the University of Nebraska and a masters degree in health administration from the University of Missouri-Columbia.

Michael W. Murphy, CPA, has been President and CEO of Sharp HealthCare since June 1996. Sharp is the largest health system and the largest private-sector employer in San Diego, with four acute care hospitals, four specialty hospitals, three medical groups, and a health plan. Mr. Murphy currently serves on a number of healthcare boards and committees throughout the country and, locally, is vice-chairman of the board of directors of the San Diego Regional Chamber of Commerce and the California Association of Hospitals and Health Systems Board of Trustees. He also actively supports a number of San Diego organizations such as the American Heart Association, MS Society, American Cancer Society, and the Union of Pan Asian Communities.

Detlev H. (Herb) Smaltz, PhD, FHIMSS, CHE, CKM, has a dual appointment at the University of Alabama at Birmingham (UAB) Health System, a $1 billion-plus academic center, where he is an Associate Professor in the Health Informatics Program and also serves as the Chief Technology Officer. Prior to his appointment at UAB, Dr. Smaltz was the first-ever Chief Knowledge Officer for the U.S. Air Force Medical Service, a $6.2 billion globally distributed integrated delivery system. In previous positions, he served as the CIO for a 20-bed community hospital, a 301-bed academic medical center, a 5-state region, and a 7-country region. Dr. Smaltz is a Diplomate in the American College of Healthcare Executives and a Fellow in HIMSS. He served on the HIMSS Board of Directors from 2002 to 2005 and as Vice-Chair of the same board from 2004 to 2005. He earned an MBA from the Ohio State University and a PhD from Florida State University.

William A. Spooner has been CIO for the past 8 of his 25 years at Sharp HealthCare in San Diego. He has led an aggressive IT effort that has placed Sharp on the Hospitals and Health Networks 100 Most Wired list for all six years since the list was established. Sharp has been an early leader in EDI development among its payers and providers. Sharp was also recognized as an early adopter for its leading edge consumer Web site. Mr. Spooner is a member of the Healthcare Information Systems Executive Association (HISEA), the College of Healthcare Information Management Executives (CHIME) and HIMSS. He is currently serving on the CHIME Board of Trustees. He has presented the Sharp model at several industry conferences.

Rulon F. Stacey, PhD, is CEO of Poudre Valley Health System, a five-hospital system based in Fort Collins, Colorado. In 1999 Dr. Stacey received the Robert S. Hudgens Award from the American College of Healthcare Executives as the "Young Healthcare Executive of the Year." In 1992, Dr. Stacey was named one of 12 executives under age 40 "who have taken considerable strides to improve the cost, access and overall quality of healthcare delivery in the United States" by Modern Healthcare *magazine. Dr. Stacey holds a bachelor of science degree in economics, a masters degree in health administration from Brigham Young University, and a doctor of philosophy in health policy from the University of Colorado.*

Michael R. Waldrum, MD, MS, has been the Chief Operating Officer of UAB Health System since December 2004. Prior to that he was the CIO of UAB Health System since June 1999 and provided leadership and oversight of all Health System Information Services (HSIS) activities and coordinated IT and IM strategies for the entities of the health system. Prior to becoming the CIO, he was the Medical Director for HSIS, where he was responsible for directing strategic projects such as Physician Order Entry and Clinical Document Access (CDA). In addition, Dr. Waldrum also continues to practice medicine within the UAB Health System and is the Medical Director for the UAB Hospital Medical Intensive Care Unit. Dr. Waldrum received his medical degree from the University of Alabama School of Medicine. He completed his residency in internal medicine at the Mayo Clinic and then returned to UAB to train in pulmonary and critical care medicine. He also has an MS in epidemiology from the Harvard School of Public Health.

References

1. Hayden F: A Mars/Pluto Relationship. *Optimize Magazine.* 2002; Issue 22. Available at http://www.optimizemag.com.
2. King J: Chasm Closer: The CIO/CEO Gap Still Dogs IS. *Computerworld.* 1995; 29(21); 84–85.
3. Klug L. Hatred: An Update (CIO-CEO Relationships). *Forbes.* 1996; 158(8); 100–104.
4. The Certification Commission for Healthcare Information Technology. Available at www.cchit.org. Accessed December 5, 2004.

CHAPTER 8

Data Rich, Information Poor: Building a Knowledge-Enabled Organization

Detlev H. (Herb) Smaltz, PhD, FHIMSS, CHE, CKM, and
Terence T. Cunningham, III, MHA, FACHE

At 7 a.m., Sam Weatherspoon arrived in the hospital's executive offices and turned on his computer. The screen flashed with new e-mails. He learned that during the evening the emergency department went on ambulance diversion. The blood bank there has 65 units of "A" positive blood. The census report shows 26 patients in critical care beds. Eight cardiac catherizations and 40 surgical cases are scheduled for today. The average accounts receivable is 72 days. Patient satisfaction scores are now 65% satisfactory and the nosocomial infection rate is 2.4%.

For the first ten minutes of the day, Sam is in information overload. His computer screen provides a wealth of data, but he feels information poor and frustrated. All of the above statistics could be good or bad news, depending upon this particular hospital's operation. The data beg the question: What really is happening in the Emergency Room, Intensive Care Units, Surgical Scheduling, Blood Bank, Bed Control, Cath Lab, AR Collections, Patient Advocate's Office, and the Infection Control Office, and how is the IT office helping Sam make informed decisions? Do the numbers show an improving situation or do the indicators illustrate a worsening problem? The computer has not given Sam benchmarks to use for comparison.

Later that same morning during Sam's meeting with the COO, they reviewed their efforts to improve the operating margin. The COO commented that they still could not get good data on costs and revenue by clinical service line or by physician. In addition, a myriad of issues plagued their efforts to improve the revenue cycle. The two major reasons that claims wound up in the error queue were the lack of a diagnosis on orders and missing documentation to support the claim.

Sam wondered why they had these problems since they had recently implemented an integrated suite of clinical and financial applications. The COO noted that the suite should have corrected these issues.

When Sam asked why they still had these problems, the COO was at a loss to explain.

The situation at Ingalls, Sam's hospital, is not unlike that in many other healthcare service delivery organizations that have invested in clinical and business IT without gaining full value of these investments. While a temptation exists to hold healthcare software application vendors responsible for this situation, the lion's share of the responsibility actually falls squarely in the purview of the healthcare organization itself. *The senior executives of these organizations have invested in technology without also putting in place the strategy, people, processes and structuring arrangements to leverage their investments in IT.* In short, they have invested in building an IT infrastructure but never really focused on also building an information management (IM) "info" structure—an information infrastructure focused on embedding, or baking-in, decision-quality information into all of the healthcare organization's key processes.

BEYOND IT INFRASTRUCTURE TO IM INFOSTRUCTURE

Just as a home builder needs the architect's design in order to successfully achieve the architect's vision for the home, the CEO needs to consider what sort of design is in place at his/her organization (if any) to achieve the vision of fully leveraging the vast quantities of data, information and knowledge that reside within and beyond his/her organization. Figure 8-1 presents a high level design framework for building a knowledge-enabled organization.

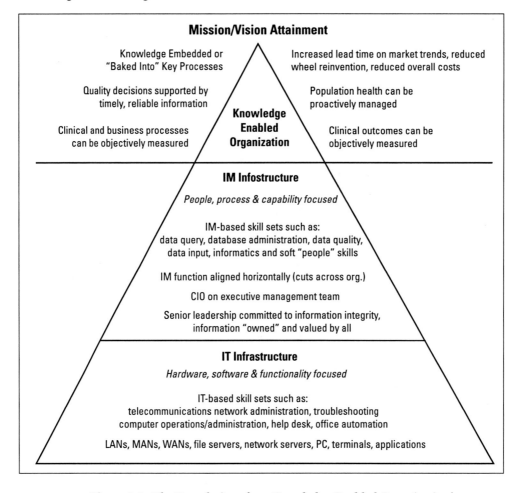

Figure 8-1. The Foundations for a Knowledge-Enabled Organization[1]

While there doesn't seem to be one universally accepted name for the IT department, recently the term "information management/information technology," or IM/IT for short, has become popular to mean all things dealing with information systems. The authors like this term because it addresses both the foundational aspects of building a knowledge-enabled organization (i.e., the IT infrastructure) as well as the higher-order functions that need to be explicitly designed into organizations (i.e., the IM "infostructure") in order to be successful.

Today, virtually every CEO, COO and CFO in the country is acutely aware of the importance of building a reliable IT infrastructure. This involves building reliable local area and wide area networks, ensuring that there is adequate power back-up capability for the computer room(s), ensuring that adequate file servers and data storage devices exist, and ensuring that adequate technical staff are in place to maintain the IT infrastructure.

The technical skill sets that are important to sustaining a solid IT infrastructure include telecommunications and network administration and troubleshooting, computer operations and administration, end-user/help desk support, functional applications support and office automation support. The authors cannot think of an organization that has not invested in, and continues to invest in renewing its IT infrastructure. Almost universally, this function—managing the IT infrastructure, or managing outsourced partners that accomplish the day-to-day functions associated with managing the IT infrastructure—is the responsibility of the organization's IT department, typically the CIO or the Chief Technology Officer (CTO).

On the other hand, fully leveraging the data and information that is generated by the various functional applications in place at organizations is akin to searching for the Holy Grail. Few healthcare organizations have, with forethought, built an *enterprise* information management capability. Generally, clinical or business departments within the healthcare organization have, over time, hired on expertise for department-specific data analysis, data query, data reporting, data aggregation, data quality, and the like. As a result, there tend to be pockets of expertise that understand slices of the enterprise's data and information, but no single person or department that fully understands all of the enterprise's data/information and how to use it cross-functionally to better inform executive decision making.

A classic sign that an organization suffers from a lack of IM capability can be ascertained by witnessing the various departmental presentations for new projects or acquisitions during the annual budget/capital review process. Does each department use a different figure for even simple, common data points such as the number of operating beds at the facility, the number of FTEs at the facility, annual revenues from the most recent fiscal year, and so forth? If different departments are not even using the same figures for things as simple as these, how can a CEO or a board of directors be assured that the projects being presented to them have been adequately analyzed using the definitive data and information sources available within the enterprise?

In order to overcome the myopic effects of the islands or pockets of IM capability within your organization, a deliberate, explicit commitment to build the IM infostructure depicted in Figure 8-1 is suggested. Clearly IT is a necessary—but not sufficient— tool for building a knowledge-enabled organization. By systemically and explicitly putting in place organizational forms and functions that focus on both building and maintaining the IT infrastructure as well as the IM infostructure depicted in Figure 8-1, organizations create the prerequisites for transforming their organization into a truly knowledge-enabled organization—one that can leverage its full complement of data, information and knowledge on the important strategic and tactical decisions it faces on its journey toward mission and vision attainment.

CHALLENGES OF BUILDING A KNOWLEDGE-ENABLED ORGANIZATION

Many information-intensive industries clearly demonstrate, via their organizational and process structuring arrangements, an understanding of the difference between IT and IM. However, more than a few healthcare organizations still seem largely unaware of the distinction. For many in healthcare service delivery, IM or IT is "the systems department." IM is not, in many cases, a comprehensive, enterprisewide, executive management responsibility and, in organizations where it is an executive level responsibility, it is largely shared among the COO, CFO, CIO, the CMO and others. Although there is a great deal of talk about the importance of IM in the healthcare industry, the lack of structures, processes, and incentives to support true enterprise IM indicates that more action needs to be taken. Despite inroads made to the healthcare sector during the late 1980s and early 1990s by the quality movement, with its process measurement/information focus, the "reinvention of the corporation" is ongoing.

One criticism of many healthcare organizations is that they remain highly compartmentalized and that the various departments and entities do not work together well enough to effectively use the IT infrastructure in place. At the risk of oversimplifying and generalizing, we note that the information systems office/department of organizations are known for focusing on offering technical solutions and keeping networks operating efficiently—in short, it has been primarily IT-focused. Furthermore, at the hospital and clinic level (where the actual healthcare "rubber meets the road"), CIOs have historically not been empowered or resourced to integrate and optimize the processes that provide and distribute information. The result is that healthcare organizations view the IM/IT department as a provider of faster/better hardware, infrastructure, and capacity to communicate. This view has been accepted and promulgated throughout the industry for years. While healthcare organizations continue to excel at building and renewing the IT infrastructure, decision makers throughout the enterprise remain skeptical, like Sam in our example, about the value gained from IT investments.

To be fully understood, these points require further clarification. Few within healthcare would dispute the value gained from IT investments to support what is largely transaction-level data processing for acute/episodic care decision making, despite some recent high-profile medical error/medication error cases. Many integrated hospital information systems provide excellent patient appointing, admissions, discharges, transfers, ancillary test ordering, and results reporting in support of physician decisions relating to acute/episodic care. Organizations such as Partners Healthcare System [2] in Boston and the Department of Defense[3] have implemented healthcare information systems with "baked in" knowledge alerting physicians and other caregivers about drug-

drug interactions, drug-food interactions, and drug-patient (allergies) interactions, which have improved quality and reduced cost for these health systems. Indeed, increasingly commercial-off-the-shelf (COTS) healthcare applications are either offering such baked-in information and/or knowledge or are making it increasingly easier to plug third-party knowledge bases into existing healthcare applications. These are certainly important elements of building a knowledge-enabled organization. However, the focus of this chapter is on leveraging the sea of data that your transaction processing systems typically generate as a by product, which then sits in vertical silos inaccessible to many of the decision-makers, like Sam, in today's typical healthcare organization.

Most organizations would agree that realization of investments in IT fall short when attempting to truly assess population health, to manage disease processes within that population, to analyze variation in practice patterns among physicians, to determine the efficacy of long-term health promotion programs, to gauge the benefit of outsourcing to other healthcare providers, or, in some cases, to gain a true picture of their own organization's performance in spite of the mounds of data available to do so. Interestingly, the IT functionality (for the most part) currently exists to create these capabilities. However, responsibility for ensuring that the IT assets are used effectively and efficiently has primarily fallen on users who, in general, know little about the systems or their full capabilities (beyond what they need to know to accomplish transactions within their responsibility), making it impossible to achieve full realization of IT benefits. While some might call for more training or for vendors to make information systems easier to use (which certainly is beneficial), *organizations cannot avoid investing in people, processes and capabilities that are expressly focused on leveraging enterprise-wide data, information and knowledge (i.e., an IM infostructure), if they want to truly achieve and sustain superior clinical and business results.*

BEST PRACTICES IN BUILDING A KNOWLEDGE-ENABLED ORGANIZATION

There are a number of characteristics of organizations that operate as a knowledge-enabled organization—organizations that have built on their IT infrastructure and also invested in building a robust IM "infostructure." These organizations have systematically and explicitly put in place a number of IM infostructure-building activities such as:

- Strategic data mapping (explicitly linking data/information needs to strategic goals/ objectives)
- Enterprise performance measurement
  - Data warehousing
  - Digital dashboards
  - Central support for data query and analysis
  - Data mining
- Knowledge management
- Web portals

Best Practice 1: Strategic Data Mapping

Most organizations take the time to periodically think through their identity: what it is, whom it serves and what it wants to become in the future. Generally, organizations document this in the form of a strategic plan. *Amazingly, after taking the time to document its mission, vision and goals, more than a few organizations fall short of mapping out an explicit roadmap for achieving its documented strategic goals and objectives.* The strategic plan in these organizations serves as a decorative artifact that is displayed prominently on executive shelves, where it effectively sucks up dust until the next JCAHO or similar audit when it is dusted off and rolled out in all its majesty to impress inspectors who presumably cannot tell whether or not the proverbial emperor is wearing any clothes. In short, it does little to serve as an active tool to continually guide organizational decision making up and down the enterprise.

Strategic data mapping refers to the practice of *explicitly* identifying key information that is needed at the various levels of the organization, and particularly at the executive level, in order to effectively assess how well the organization is doing with respect to achieving the goals and objectives laid out in its strategic plan. While a seemingly obvious step, many organizations write a strategic plan and then do not set in place performance measurement activities that are fully in line with that strategic plan. To be sure, standard measures exist for every organization like days accounts receivable or adjusted bed days, but few organizations fully measure, in a systematic, consistent manner, *all* of the objectives and goals that have been articulated in its strategic plan.

Strategic data mapping can be accomplished either as a distinct extension of plain ole' vanilla strategic planning or can be accomplished in conjunction with various frameworks such as John Rockart's critical success factor (CSF) methodology,[4] Norton and Kaplan's balanced scorecard methodology,[5] or the European Foundation for Quality Management's Excellence Model,[6] to name but a few. The authors used the CSF approach, as early as 1990, to build an enterprise strategic data map to identify organizational blind spots and take steps to explicitly put in place means of measuring the areas, that to date, had not been measured. *Regardless of which framework it uses, the critical point here is that the organization takes the time to identify, at a minimum, all of the data/information items needed to continually assess how well it is doing with respect to achieving its strategic goals and objectives.* See Figure 8-2 for a high-level process for accomplishing a strategic data map and Appendix 8-1 for a mini-case study of how Brigham and Women's Hospital CIO Sue Shade used the balanced scorecard approach.

Once an organization has done that, it is ready to create an enterprise performance measurement capability. Ideally, this is done by offloading data from transaction processing systems onto what is known as a data warehouse or data mart that can be used exclusively for organizational performance assessments at all levels of the organization (office, department, branch, division, unit, enterprise), without negatively impacting transaction processing systems. In the process of putting a data warehouse in place, it will be essential to also build in the people and processes to explicitly address the data quality problems that an organization is sure to find as data is pulled from a myriad of source systems into a single data warehouse.

Steps to create an organizational strategic data map:

Executive Staff/Board of Director Actions:
1. Ideally, convene the executive staff and board of an organization to an offsite location. Start by reviewing the organization's strategic plan to ensure it continues to be an accurate reflection of the organization's mission, vision, goals and objectives.
2. Assuming it is, start with each goal/objective and determine the 1 to 3 critical success factors that must happen in order for the organization to meet that goal/objective.
3. For each of these critical success factors, determine the data needs in order to assess them. Do not limit yourself to only data that you know you now collect. The goal here is to simply identify all of the data you need to assess performance with respect to the critical success factors you have identified.

Organization Data Gurus' Actions:
4. Once the executive management team and board of directors has completed steps 1 to 3, convene a "data guru" panel/committee made up of your organization's data experts to identify specific data elements and the specific information system(s) where the data reside.
5. For identified data needs where there currently is no data collected, have the panel/committee recommend potential means of collecting this previously uncollected data.
6. Publish the strategic data map as a follow-on effort to all future organizational strategic planning efforts. That way you are continually reinforcing your organizational commitment to building an end-to-end strategy-to-data linkage and, by extension, a key component of your IM infostructure.

Figure 8-2. A Generic Strategic Data Mapping Process

Enterprise Performance Measurement

While organizations don't necessarily have to use an enterprise performance measurement framework, many organizations find them useful. Indeed, particularly organizations that have already invested in putting in place such frameworks as Kaplan & Morton's Balanced Scorecard or the European Foundation for Quality Management's Excellence Model, to name but a few, will find the strategic data mapping exercise useful in creating an instant blueprint for building an enterprise performance measurement capability regardless of the performance measurement framework employed. In fact, CEOs and scholars alike lament that many organizations continue to fall short of identifying measures for continually assessing goals and objectives[7] even if they are using frameworks such as those noted above.[8] The most likely cause for this is that *many organizations accomplish steps 1 to 3 in the strategic data mapping process outlined in Figure 8-2, but few actually mandate the detailed level work by data gurus outlined in steps 4 to 6 to first identify the exact data elements in the exact information systems that will provide them with strategic feedback they need, and second to turn that data, residing in a myriad of systems, into useful, timely, appropriately refreshed information to continually assess organizational performance.*

If an organization accomplishes strategic data mapping, it links the critical data/information needed to assess *all* of the strategic goals and objectives that it has identified and, by extension, it will have in place the fundamentals for enterprise performance measurement. Within the area of enterprise performance measurement there are two additional key best practices with respect to building enterprise performance measurement capability. The first is to pull transaction level data off into a data warehouse whose primary function is to assist the entire organization with analyses and decision support. The second is to build a digital dashboard that draws from the data warehouse to continually assess the data/information identified in the strategic data mapping effort.

Best Practice 2: Data Warehousing

If an organization does not already have a data warehouse, or even if it does, one of the first things to be discovered upon completing the strategic data mapping effort is just how disparate and far flung key data really are—and not just any data. This is the data that the organization has identified as critical to being able to continually assess progress toward the organization's strategic goals and objectives. The organization will find that some of it resides in the patient registry system, some in the laboratory system, some in stand-alone data bases created on individuals' PCs, some in a strategic partner's systems, and the like. Furthermore, the organization's staff will inform leadership that accomplishing analyses on these transaction-processing systems has a negative impact on their primary transaction-based functions. In other words, if an organization wants to conduct a study to reduce laboratory costs on the laboratory system proper, the act of analyzing the data negatively impacts the performance of the lab system, and lab results reporting and subsequent clinical intervention will be delayed pending the data analysis.

Also, an organization ideally does not want to require all of its analysts to understand the intricacies of multiple disparate database structures and file and table structures (the guts of these systems' databases) in order to accomplish the analyses. Ideally, an organization wants to be able to access critical strategic data in one place for one-stop shopping when it comes to enterprise performance measurement. Enter the enterprise data warehouse.

Enterprise data warehouses essentially provide a homogeneous location for the data that heterogeneously resides in your various information systems. Since the focus in this text is executive management, it will not go into the nuts and bolts of building enterprise data warehouses. Once executive resolve is in place to focus efforts on building and maintaining an enterprise data warehouse, the CIO should be able to manage the building of an enterprise data warehouse relatively easily, or oversee such an effort by a third party vendor specializing in data warehousing.

The way an enterprise data warehouse typically functions is that data collected from the main transaction-based systems (appointing and scheduling, laboratory, pharmacy, etc.) is copied over to the data warehouse for use in organizational analyses and performance measurement activities. Once in the data warehouse, it serves as the one-stop shopping for management engineering studies, operations research studies, clinical process studies, and other decision support processes. Most recently, enterprise data warehouses have enabled the new field of data mining (large variable data set correlation and associative studies). This will be covered in more detail in subsequent sections. In addition to serving as the nexus for analyst and informaticist studies in your organization, the enterprise data warehouse also usefully serves as the feeder system for executive digital dashboards, where the information identified in the strategic data mapping process can be cogently displayed for easy reference and assessment. Digital dashboards will also be covered in more detail in a subsequent section.

Some additional considerations that executives should discuss when building enterprise data warehouses include, but are not limited to, synchronization, access and security, and data accuracy/quality/reconciliation activities.

Data Warehouse Design Considerations: Data Synchronization (Real-Time or Near Real-Time)

To be sure, where the "rubber meets the road" for all of an organization's clinical information-based processes is typically in the front-line primary transaction-based information systems so they typically are real-time. So the authors want to make a clear distinction here between those front-line transaction processing systems (ADT, lab, rad, pharmacy, and the like) and your enterprise data warehouse, which, as we described earlier, basically receives data from these front-line transaction systems for later use to aid analyses and decision support. Without a doubt, if cost were no object, all healthcare organizations would want to have real-time data available in their enterprise data warehouse to assist decision support and organizational performance measurement processes. But cost is an object, and therefore some level below real-time is usually more cost effective with minimal impacts on management decision quality.

Many organizations find that for many processes, daily, weekly or even monthly data synchronization is effective for performance measurement and management decision support. Does the organization really need immediate downloads to the enterprise data warehouse for *all/any* of its data? Clearly, if processes are identified in the strategic data map that are more time sensitive (practice pattern trends, epidemiological surveillance, and the like), the organization may want to set these data items to update at intervals throughout the day. For others, such as access to care metrics, wellness and health promotion metrics, disease management, and the like, daily, weekly, or even monthly downloads are quite adequate, depending on the specific process. The point is that the frequency of data synchronization from your main transaction-based systems to your enterprise data warehouse should be dictated by the sensitivity of each data element's ability to provide time-sensitive management actionable insight to your organization's key processes.

Data Warehouse Design Considerations: Access and Security

Again, since the focus on this chapter is at the executive level of an organization, a detailed, blow-by-blow Privacy Act/HIPAA implementation plan is not warranted here and is readily available in a multitude of publications. Organizations have no choice but to implement Privacy Act/HIPAA-compliant processes. Rather, this chapter focuses on the access and security considerations that should be assessed when putting an enterprise data warehouse in place, with the assumption that the organization's privacy officer and/or CIO must build in Privacy Act and HIPAA compliance.

While data warehouses are essential to continual enterprise performance measurement capabilities and building the IM infostructure, they create new challenges with respect to access and security. On the one hand, all staff who need to accomplish analyses and support decision processes should have access to the enterprise data warehouse. On the other hand, strong federal legislation (e.g., Privacy Act, HIPAA) is in place to ensure that only authorized access is granted to patient-identifiable information. Unfortunately, the explosion of access to detailed sensitive information has not always been accompanied by a general awareness of the laws and rules governing its accumulation, handling, use, protection and release. A wide range of improper practices is continually uncovered: patient sensitive information is being accessed by individuals who do not have an official need to know; data are being stored on unsecured media and/or unsecure systems; databases subject to the Privacy Act/HIPAA are not adhering to the provisions of the Acts; passwords are being shared; and sensitive data about identified patients are being provided for research when aggregate data would suffice.

These are but a few of the common improper practices that need to be explicitly addressed when building/maintaining an enterprise data warehouse. Bottom line, an organization really needs to explicitly review its data/information access policies and processes to ensure that (1) staff has the ability to accomplish effective performance measurement and affect change; and (2) safeguards are in place to prevent unauthorized access to the same data/information.

Data Warehouse Design Considerations: Data Quality Assurance Activities

While few executives ever, in any industry or field, enjoy 100% reliability with respect to the information available to them at the point of a decision, the development of an enterprise data warehouse requires an explicit ongoing focus on data quality assurance. Without a doubt, every healthcare executive ideally would like to have consistent access to perfectly accurate data all of the time. With issues such as human error at the point of data input into the front-line transaction-based systems and synchronization (discussed previously), there will always be some level of data that is either dated or not error-free. The key with respect to data warehousing is to have an explicit process in place to address data quality assurance and seek to continually minimize data inaccuracies. To effectively accomplish this really requires developing a data quality culture throughout the entire organization.

An obsessive commitment to data quality assurance is a fundamental building block of an IM infostructure, and by extension, a knowledge-enabled organization. In the IT infrastructure-centric model, the focus was on fielding information systems, training users, and then essentially leaving them alone to attempt their data analyses. Without a sound understanding of the dynamics involved in ensuring data validity and the methods of extracting data from disparate systems, users produced suboptimal data analyses that formed the basis of business process decision-making. *In the IM infostructure-centric model, quality decisions are informed by numerous full-time staff that fully understands the sources of data, its validity and how to extract it. This has an orders-of-magnitude leveraging effect on an organization's knowledge workers to objectively and rigorously assess their processes and strategies.*

Besides committing dedicated resources to the pursuit of data quality, organizations must also recognize that data quality cannot be centrally controlled, though a cell of individuals focused on continually assessing organizational data and pointing out potential data quality problems can be centralized. However, to have an effective enterprise performance measurement capability, data quality must become the mantra of everyone in the organization in order to ensure a solid information foundation for decision-making. Particularly important are data input sites to an organization's transaction-based information systems, where most data quality problems originate. Because the data in a data warehouse originates in these front-end transaction-based systems, organizations will want to correct data quality problems at the source system rather than once it is already in the data warehouse.

From a human resources perspective, it is important to recognize that many organizations in healthcare entrust a most important function (i.e., data entry to the information repositories that will form the basis of enterprise decision-making) to individuals in jobs that are among the lowest paid and often seen as least desirable. To overcome the natural complacency that these jobs induce, organizations must focus attention on these prime sites of data quality failure and implement effective rewards and incentives to change behavior in a positive manner. Because all information systems with login-password control can track which user is inputting data, it becomes easy for a central data quality function to identify consistently solid data input from problematic data input and via training, rewards and incentives minimize data quality problems that occur at the front end.

Best Practice 3: Digital Dashboards

While the data warehouse serves as the one-stop shopping for all of the organization's data analysts, it also serves as the source for digital dashboards. These are report card-like digital displays that executive management can use to continually assess organizational performance on key metrics. For organizations that accomplish strategic data mapping (described earlier), actually depicting the strategic goals and objectives on the digital dashboard is a reinforcing means of communicating to the entire organization why the measures in the dashboard are important.

Typically, digital dashboards are Internet/Web-based and provide layered views of performance measures. At the executive level view, the authors suggest no more than 20 to 30 key high level measures are presented that cover the waterfront in continually communicating to senior executives how the organization is doing with respect to stated strategic goals and objectives. Just below the executive layer, world-class digital dashboards have the ability for middle managers or inquisitive senior executives to drill down to assess a host of feeder processes. In other words, for some organizational strategic goals, there may be four or five submeasures that are used to create one executive level measure.

World-class digital dashboards present information with legends or footnotes to explain how certain information was derived or calculated and provide a point of contact so that the user can telephone or e-mail to obtain needed clarification. For example, is percent bed occupancy a calculation of the number of patients and infants in beds divided by the number of licensed beds, beds physically set up, or staffed beds? There are several different answers to this one question depending on definition of terms and the method of calculation. The information must be presented in an easy to understand format and, when appropriate, with an accompanying text to help avoid misunderstandings.

In addition, world-class digital dashboards also provide context and/or benchmarks whenever possible. One of the most frustrating features of reviewing rows and columns of data and graphical charts is not being able to quickly understand what ideas are being transmitted. The number "65 units of A+ blood" used in the first paragraph of this chapter means nothing to most people who do not work in that hospital's blood bank. If that hospital routinely uses 80 units of A+ blood daily, the 65 units figure would prompt the staff to take actions such as delaying some elective surgery cases, asking the metropolitan area blood bank if a supplemental delivery of blood can be made, and so forth. If that hospital routinely uses only 40 units of A+ blood, the 65-unit figure is good news and additional follow-up action is probably not necessary.

The design of the computer templates and screens should include the needs of the users who will review the information. Putting a benchmark along side the actual data provides for a very helpful comparison that allows the managers to quickly review the information and manage by exception. A benchmark can be a national or local standard, a historical number, a running 12-month average, or other predetermined calculations. While many of the common healthcare information systems vendor's clinical applications have built in clinical benchmarks and alerts, many business systems do not require local processes to set them up (for the example above, to show the average daily volume of blood products consumed, adjusted for any seasonal or other cyclical anomalies).

In addition, world-class digital dashboards provide subscription services or "push" reporting whereby an executive, middle manager, physician, nurse, or any member of the organization, can subscribe to key measures and each time they are updated in the data warehouse and digital dashboard, a report of the measure of interest is generated and sent in an e-mail to the subscribing individual. That way, the individual doesn't have to go to the digital dashboard until something of interest to her has changed. An example of a digital dashboard can be found in Figures 8-3 and 8-4.

The digital dashboard depicted is for a large geographically distributed integrated delivery system. Figure 8-3 depicts one of the integrated delivery system's key strategic performance measures (equivalent outpatient visits) for one of its regions. Note the ability to subscribe via the "push" reports feature. In addition, this digital dashboard has drill-down capability such that when a user clicks on one of the region's large outpatient clinics, he or she can drill down all the way to individual provider, as depicted in Figure 8-4. All of the data generated on this digital dashboard is generated from a data warehouse, which, of course, received its data from front-line transaction processing systems (like the IDS's patient appointing and scheduling application). Typically, this IDS chooses a monthly synchronization for this measure to keep costs down.

Internet or Web-based digital dashboards are powerful tools not only for communicating and continually reinforcing a strong executive message throughout the organization but also in positively changing behavior along the organization's strategic goal waterfront. *The old adage, "what gets measured gets done" holds true – even more so when everyone in the organization can see what is being done well and what is not.*

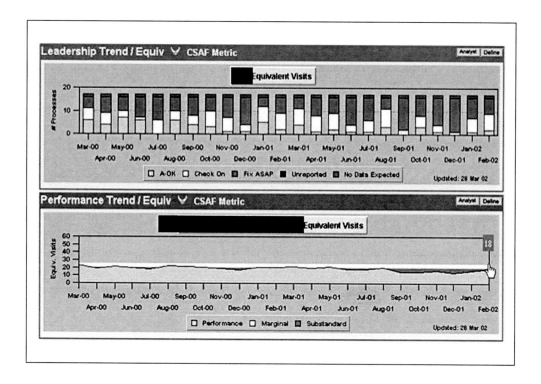

Figure 8-3. A Sample Enterprise Digital Dashboard.
(Courtesy of Lt. Col. Rick Reichard for use of the U.S. Air Force Medical Service's digital dashboard.)

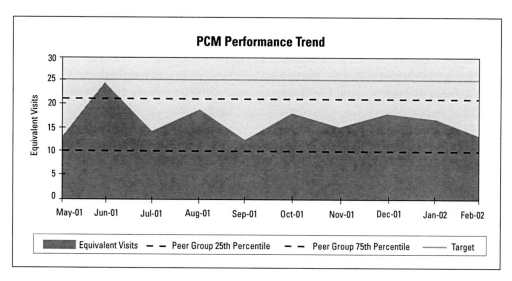

Figure 8-4. A Sample Enterprise Digital Dashboard-Drill-Down View.
(Courtesy of Lt. Col. Rick Reichard for use of the U.S. Air Force Medical Service's digital dashboard.)

Though some organizations may want to draw the line with respect to who has visibility into which measures and to what level, organization level or business unit level measures are most powerful in motivating positive action if they are visible to all. And individual level measures can be powerful if each individual can see their performance with respect to the norms of their peers. But without a doubt, digital dashboards are much more than information tools—they are an incredibly effective communication medium and strategy reinforcing tool.

Best Practice 4: Central Support for Data Query, Analysis, Informatics and Decision Support

A number of healthcare organizations recognize the value of centralized approaches to data management and query. They have created management engineering, operations research or decision support departments whose function is to serve as the central support for data query and first-line analyses. Others may have created such departments but find it useful to have multiple decision support departments (e.g., business decision support department and a separate clinical decision support department). Still other healthcare service delivery organizations have a totally decentralized approach to data query and analysis.

While not obvious to most, the costs to the organization increase with the level of decentralization. While highly specialized human resources in, say, clinical care, may be better suited to forming clinical process questions, they may be used suboptimally in writing complex queries or other data "geek" tasks, when their primary function should be patient care or some other business function. Clearly this drives up costs. In addition, it makes for a Tower of Babel–Wild, Wild West situation when department analyses are used to inform a board on investment or strategic decisions. One department may use one set of assumptions for an analyses while another may use a different assumption. One department may use only staffed beds when calculating a measure while another may use all beds for the same measure. In short, the more hands in the cookie jar, the more chaotic an organization's analysis capability becomes, ultimately frustrating quality decision-making and the organization's strategy.

The first author of this chapter initiated a pilot project in a former organization whereby a regional data cell provides data query and analysis support to seven hospitals and clinics in the region. Business managers, group practice managers, clinical staff, and the like pose business/clinical questions of the central data cell which then determines exactly what the requestor is looking for and provides it to them in the format desired (whether as a graph, a chart, a spreadsheet or a database).

Initial findings indicate a number of positive outcomes from this pilot. First, individuals who previously spent part of their work day learning how to do such things as writing structured query language (SQL) queries, or learning a particular data analysis tool, now spend their time thinking about the business and clinical processes that they are trying to improve. The "grunt" data query and analysis work is left to centralized expertise that already has these skills in place. So, in short, FTEs are working on tasks in their job descriptions as opposed to doing "grunt" level data geek activities better suited to experts. Second, these seven hospitals and clinics previously had 10.5 FTEs accomplishing these "grunt" level duties which now three FTEs provide centrally, a savings, in this example, of 7.5 FTEs. Finally, by making centralized requests, the central headquarters function learns about common questions being asked at the facility level. For common questions, the central cell typically provides the same data that one facility asked for, for all of the hospitals and clinics on the central digital dashboard and via push reports. Push reports are simply reports that are sent out, often via e-mail, to individuals that have expressed a need to have operational metrics at each hospital and clinic.

If a healthcare delivery organization is a stand-alone entity, centralized approaches may be prescribed as well, if the organization has multiple departments that work independently to accomplish "grunt" level data queries and reports.

It is important to point out that these central data support cells in no way take the place of clinical and business process subject matter experts which continue to function in their respective primary roles. What they do is ensure that these often highly compensated clinical and business process staff are focused on their primary duty rather than also continually having to learn how to be a data "geek." Instead they formulate business questions or clinical questions that data experts provide to support services to serve them in a manner that best suites the clinicians or business manager's needs.

Best Practice 5: Data Mining

By using data mining techniques, organizations that have invested in building an enterprise data warehouse and that have a central or core business unit focused on data query/analysis/reporting have the ability to discover a host of non-intuitive opportunities (e.g., revenue cycle compression, revenue generation, cost avoidance, quality improvement). Recently the Florida Hospital in Orlando won an award for its use of data mining techniques via its enterprise data warehouse to discover a number of non-obvious revenue generation, cost avoidance and quality enhancing opportunities. More and more healthcare organizations are recognizing that enterprise data warehouses are essential to enable them to discover potential areas for improvement that have a positive impact on the bottom line, patient safety and quality.

While the best practices outlined in the enterprise performance measurement sections of this chapter do not necessarily need to be built in sequential fashion, in order to pursue data mining techniques, an organization must have first developed a cadre of data "geeks," affectionately called so, who have a thorough understanding of the organization's data. These are the same people who assisted in steps 4 to 6 of the strategic data mapping exercise, helped in building and maintaining the enterprise data warehouse, and who staff the central decision support, informatics, or data analysis support department. In addition, someone with either an extensive background in statistics or computational mathematics or both becomes important.

Data mining can be used to build predictive models, for trend analysis, for business intelligence, for hidden associations and correlations and a host of other organization leveraging activities.

Knowledge Management

It is beyond the scope of this chapter to fully cover the topic of knowledge management. The first author is presently working on an entire book on the topic of applying knowledge management in healthcare organizations. Furthermore, from a Maslow's hierarchy of needs perspective, few healthcare organizations have mastered the lower level needs of leveraging their data and information (which this chapter primarily focuses on). However, a brief overview of how knowledge management can be applied to healthcare organizations is warranted.

While a seemingly proper label for the practice of explicitly and deliberately building, renewing, and applying relevant intellectual assets to maximize an enterprise's effectiveness,[9] knowledge management or KM is a relatively misunderstood practice within the healthcare industry. Simply put, it seeks to leverage as much of the information and knowledge that exists within and beyond an organization. This knowledge can either be in explicit form (such as in databases, spreadsheets, presentation slides, or documents or other media) or in tacit form (such as the "know-how" in an individual's head). The task of knowledge managers is to explicitly and deliberately build the organizational processes and toolset that bring this knowledge asset to bear on the thousands of tactical and strategic decisions that are made each day in a healthcare organization.

Sounds simple enough, right? Unfortunately, organizations typically cannot simply leapfrog to a robust knowledge management capability. Just as a house needs a foundation before it can be framed, and framing before the roof can be installed, organizations are much better poised to reap the benefits of enterprise-wide knowledge management if they have first put in place some of the enabling capabilities of an IM infostructure previously discussed.

For organizations that have built a solid IM infostructure, building a knowledge management capability is a logical next step. Knowledge management can be thought of as a capability that can either aid frontline transaction-based decision-making or can aid less time sensitive, reflective decision-making. While not intended to be an all-inclusive list, Figure 8-5 indicates some of the focal areas within the knowledge management field.

Transactional Knowledge Management	Reflective Knowledge Management
Ideally operationalized by "baking-into" clinical and administrative systems	*Ideally operationalized via enterprise Web portals/smart enterprise suites*
• Alerts, text blobs, order sets, etc. built into frontline systems	• Taxonomies/knowledge maps
• Packaged methodologies/ best practices	• Document management
• Workflow management	• Collaboration/virtual teams
	• Expert profiling/location
	• Virtual libraries/knowledge repositories
	• E-learning
	• Auto text categorization
	• Web content management

Figure 8-5. Focal Areas Within Knowledge Management

Transactional knowledge management (e.g., order sets, rules, alerts, forms, templates, text blobs, and problem-knowledge couplers) is distinguished from reflective knowledge management (e.g., online access to peer reviewed and other clinical reference materials, expertise profiling, expert/peer location management). Transactional knowledge management components are knowledge assets that are ideally built right into, or "baked into," the clinical or business process and are helpful at the point of the transaction/service. An example of this is using First Data Bank's drug-drug adverse interaction knowledge base in conjunction with an enterprises computer-based provider order entry (CPOE) system. Reflective knowledge assets are available at the time and place of the clinical encounter or business decision but are more often accessed in a reflective mode, either prospectively or retrospectively. Examples of such assets are access to peer reviewed clinical references such as MDConsult, Micromedex, OVID, and Stat!Ref, on the clinical side and access to paid subscription services like the Meta Group, Gartner Research, or HIMSS on the business side. Typically, the reflective knowledge assets are built into an enterprise intranet, Web portal or smart enterprise suite and available on all caregiver and business manager desktops.

Again, fully covering the topic of knowledge management is beyond the scope of this text, but the authors will cover the primary means that organizations are using to operationalize knowledge management practices, which is via "one-stop shopping" enterprise Web portals.

Best Practice 6: Enterprise Web Portals/Smart Enterprise Suites, or One-Stop Shopping for Data, Information, Knowledge and Applications

One of the highest leveraging best practices an organization can implement, especially if the other components of an IM infostructure have been put in place, is building an enterprise Web portal or smart enterprise suite that provides one-stop shopping to key relevant data, information and knowledge. An organization's IM/IT department, using readily available Web services technology, or via outsourcing the development to the vendor community, can build links to existing legacy systems such that the data, information, and knowledge can be wholly or partially interacted with via a single user login account using a desktop or hand-held Web browser (Figure 8-6 is a notional representation of such a Web portal).

The leveraging power of Web portals, when correctly implemented, is phenomenal. First and foremost, it provides a single login account to multiple information systems and repositories. In addition, it only provides access to the applications and or repositories based on the individual's access rights. This is a huge frustration minimizer among clinicians and significantly simplifies the security and access management process and increases productivity. Rather than having every employee's access managed via dozens of different processes (typically via the owners of the information systems that they are trying to access), an organization now has a single means of managing access to all of your information systems and repositories. Second, rather than necessitating that staff learns dozens of different applications, properly implemented Web portals or smart enterprise suites require the user to only learn the browser-based front end. This minimizes frustration, enhances productivity, and saves training dollars. Additionally, these portals can provide a conduit to customers or patients for processes that involve them (pharmacy refills, patient appointing and scheduling, chronic disease management, and the like). Finally, it provides a means to truly bring all of the data, information and knowledge resources to bear at a single point of service.

Unfortunately many organizations have allowed parallel, competing and non-federated organizational portals to proliferate, diminishing the leveraging impact of an integrated portal (either a single portal or a number of federated portals that adhere to a common governance and set of business rules to ensure their integration). For instance, human resources (HR) may have developed an HR-specific portal, the clinical area may have created another portal, and the IM/IT department, perhaps a portal for Web content and document management. Unless there is a governance structure to integrate these disparate portals, they become islands unto themselves and cannot be leveraged across the enterprise (see Chapter 1 on effective IT governance models). Such implementations vastly diminish the ability of an organization to leverage the distributed intellectual assets captured in each of these disconnected portals.

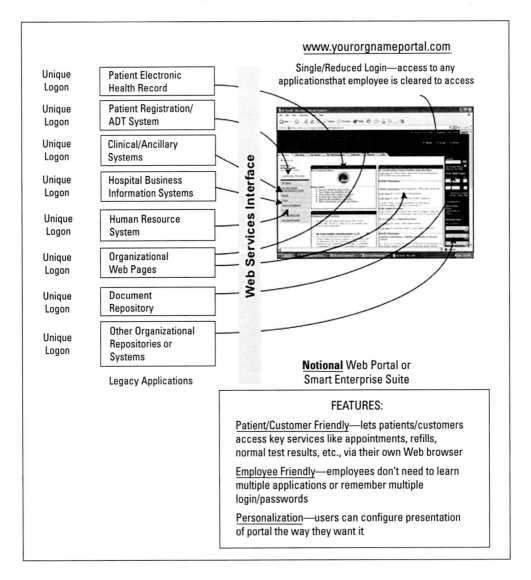

Figure 8-6. Notional Depiction of an Enterprise Web Portal or Smart Enterprise Suite

For organizations that take an integrated approach to Web portal governance and development, enterprise Web portals, or smart enterprise suites, have the ability to truly integrate the organization and provide an order of magnitude leveraging ability for healthcare organizations to better serve their communities and significantly increase their efficiency and effectiveness.

Summary

The key message for healthcare executives is that IT alone is not a proverbial silver bullet (Figure 8-7). Simply implementing technology will not automatically garner the value that is sought via these investments. Rather, *healthcare executives must deliberately and explicitly build an IM infostructure on top of the IT infrastructure if they want their organizations to become truly knowledge-enabled.* Furthermore, IM infostructures require an entirely different set of skills than do IT infrastructure building and maintenance (see Figure 8-1). It is essential that dedicated human resources not only understand the business and clinical processes of the healthcare entity but also have a comprehensive understanding of the healthcare entity's data that resides in its myriad information systems, and how to correctly extract it for business decision-making. Finally, only by putting in place both an IT infrastructure and IM infostructure can organizations begin to leverage the full complement of the distributed data, information and knowledge at its disposal and become a knowledge-enabled organization—one that not only serves the needs of its community but also one that has a competitive leg up on other organizations that have not yet invested in an IM infostructure.

Key Points for Executives

Transforming an Enterprise into a Knowledge-Enabled Organization
- IT is a necessary, but not sufficient, condition for building a knowledge-enabled organization
- In order to gain full value from IT investments, healthcare organizations must also invest in building and sustaining an IM infostructure
- Healthcare organizations that have IM infostructures are characterized by:
  - Strategic data mapping (explicitly linking data and information to its published/evolving strategic objectives and goals)
  - Engaging in enterprise performance measurement by:
    - Building and sustaining a data warehouse that
      - Possesses decision quality data
      - Is secure, yet accessible to those with a need to know
      - Is appropriately synchronized with frontline systems
    - Building and sustaining digital dashboards
    - Providing central cross-functional support for data query, analysis, informatics and decision support
    - Data mining: accomplishing large variable data set analysis to find non-intuitive trends that may represent opportunities for business/clinical process/outcome improvement
  - Knowledge management
    - Baking-in knowledge at the point of transaction (in front end IS systems)
    - Providing access to knowledge bases
    - Web portals or smart enterprise suites providing one-stop, browser-based access to all, or most, of an enterprise's information systems and other knowledge resources

---

Figure 8-7. Key Points for Creating a Knowledge-Enabled Organization

Sam was startled to realize that, although all of the management and medical staff leadership regarded data and information as an important organizational asset, Ingalls did not manage that asset comprehensively and consistently.

While he still had more to learn about information management, Sam was convinced that the organization needed to begin to pursue best practices in these areas: strategic data mapping, data warehousing, digital performance dashboards, central support and management of these activities, data mining, knowledge management, and enterprise portals.

Information management might not be as sexy as state-of-the-art IT but Sam thought it might be more important.

Detlev H. (Herb) Smaltz, PhD, FHIMSS, CHE, CKM, has a dual appointment at the University of Alabama at Birmingham (UAB) Health System, a $1 billion-plus academic center, where he is an Associate Professor in the Health Informatics Program and also serves as the Chief Technology Officer. Prior to his appointment at UAB, Dr. Smaltz was the first-ever Chief Knowledge Officer for the U.S. Air Force Medical Service, a $6.2 billion globally distributed integrated delivery system. In previous positions, he served as the CIO for a 20-bed community hospital, a 301-bed academic medical center, a 5-state region, and a 7-country region. Dr. Smaltz is a Diplomate in the American College of Healthcare Executives and a Fellow in the HIMSS. He served on the HIMSS Board of Directors from 2002 to 2005 and as Vice-Chair of the same board from 2004 to 2005. He earned an MBA from the Ohio State University and a PhD from Florida State University.

Terence T. Cunningham, III, MHA, FACHE, is the Hospital Administrator for Ben Taub General Hospital in Houston, a 650-bed academic medical center serving as the flagship teaching hospital for the Baylor College of Medicine. Ben Taub has been listed as one of the Top 100 Hospitals in the United States. Mr. Cunningham has worked with developing and managing information management activities as a senior healthcare executive for over 30 years. His assignments included the U.S. Air Force Medical Service at various hospitals and headquarters and Johns Hopkins Hospital. He has written and lectured extensively on total quality management and using continuous process improvement and continuous cost improvement in hospitals. Mr. Cunningham graduated with a BS in microbiology from California State University, Long Beach, and earned a masters degree in hospital administration from George Washington University in Washington, DC.

APPENDIX 8-1

Mini-Case Study: The Balanced Scorecard at Brigham and Women's Hospital

Brigham and Women's Hospital (BWH) is a 719-bed, nonprofit teaching affiliate of Harvard Medical School; it is also a founding member of Partners HealthCare System, an integrated healthcare delivery network. Internationally recognized as a leading academic healthcare institution, BWH is committed to excellence in patient care, medical research, and the training and education of healthcare professionals. The hospital's preeminence in all aspects of clinical care is coupled with its strength in medical research.

BWH built on its strengths by successfully pursuing a balanced scorecard initiative (BSC) on both the provider and business sides of the hospital. Like many organizations, BWH was data-rich but information-poor.

The Kaplan/Norton balanced scorecard methodology guided the development process. The "balanced" nature of the methodology resonated with BWH leadership and its desire to implement a framework that allowed a greater focus than simply financial metrics. According to the methodology, scorecards use four balanced perspectives to examine an industry or business:

- Shareholder, or financial, perspective
- External, usually customer, perspective
- Internal, typically business processes, perspective
- Knowledge and growth perspective, which normally encompasses research and development, employee growth and investment in information systems

Applying this to healthcare, BWH used the following names for the perspectives: financial health, service excellence, quality and efficiency of care, and clinical innovation. In a for-profit environment, shareholders are typically found at the top of the strategic map. Instead, Brigham and Women's Hospital placed patients (service excellence) at the top of its map.

The following steps were used in implementing each departmental scorecard:

- Establish an executive champion
- Select and educate a balanced scorecard system development group
- Develop a strategy map and strategic goals for the departments
- Inventory/brainstorm potential measures for each goal that the organization is trying to achieve
- Determine if any measures already exist and whether they can be captured electronically
- Rationalize the list of measures
- Develop measurement documentation such as definitions, data sources, frequency, and the like
- Develop data extracts (data feeds from existing source systems)
- Develop reporting specifications
- Develop the balanced scorecard reporting hierarchy and security access
- Perform data warehouse, scorecard, measurement and report programming
- Provide scorecard data for quality assurance (QA) [include steps to QA data feeds, measurement programs, supporting reports and published scorecards]
- Roll out the system; educate and train users

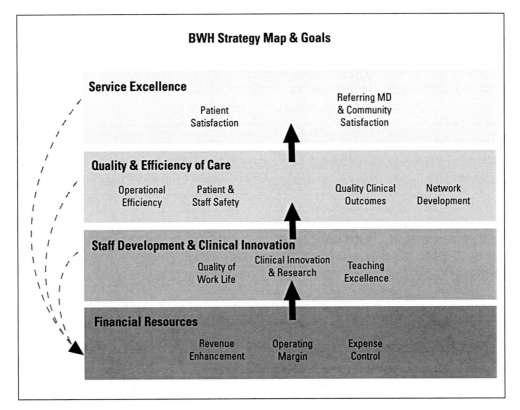

Figure 8-8. Brigham and Women's Hospital Strategy Map and Goals

Key lessons learned from this initiative include:
- Executive sponsorship and buy-in (including CEO, COO, CFO, CMO, CIO, and CNO) was key to getting the project off the ground and funded.
- CEO buy-in and use will drive success.
- VP sponsors for pilot areas need to be true advocates to ensure early wins.
- Initial reward for building and using is consolidation of existing reports and management data into "one place."
- A data warehouse that can accept key healthcare feeds, with minimal internal programming, is an essential foundation.
- Supporting reports and the level of drill-down is designed to answer the first question a user might have about a trend, not to replace source systems and reports.
- The BSC framework has been easy to explain and has been well accepted.
- The BSC has increased the sense of data transparency for users, and therefore accountability.

Last but not least, it takes time to move from the early stage of performance *measurement* to the next stage of performance *management* and then to the final stage of *strategic management.* Explicit strategies need to be developed to drive use of scorecard data and to incorporate the BSC into the strategic framework of an organization. BWH has evolved and grown through these three stages. The goals of the final stage of strategic management include:
- Board and leadership adopt BSC framework as part of strategy formulation and hospital-wide communication plan.

- Key strategic goals and measures cascade throughout all lower-level strategy maps and scorecards.
- Review of BSC goals and measuring performance is incorporated into all leadership meetings.
- Research and education goals/measures are incorporated along side strong set of clinical indicators.

ACKNOWLEDGMENTS

The authors would like to express special thanks to Sue Schade for sharing her case study on using the balanced scorecard approach within Brigham and Women's Hospital. Additionally, special thanks to Lt. Col. Rick Reichard for sharing generic screen shots of a digital dashboard for organizational performance measurement he helped develop for the U.S. Air Force Medical Service.

References

1. Smaltz D, Price R, Williamson P, Ramsaroop P: Building the Knowledge-Enabled Organization: Beyond IT Infrastructures to IM Infostructures. In Ramsaroop P, Ball M, Beaulieu D, Douglas J (eds): *Advancing Federal Sector Healthcare*. New York, NY: Springer-Verlag; 2001.
2. Davenport J, Glaser J: Just in Time Delivery Comes to Knowledge Management. *Harvard Business Review*. July 2002; 80:107–111; 126.
3. Middleton B, Christopherson G, Rocha R, Smaltz D: Knowledge Management in Clinical Systems: Principles and Pragmatics. Sept 2004; MEDINFO Panel; San Francisco, CA.
4. Rockart JF: Chief Executives Define Their Own Data Needs. *Harvard Business Review*. 1979; 57(2); 81–93.
5. Kaplan RS, Norton DP: The Balanced Scorecard. Boston MA: Harvard Business School Press; 1996.
6. European Foundation for Quality Management's Excellence Model, Available at: www.efqm.org/model_awards/model/excellence_model.htm. Accessed January 14, 2004.
7. Weston J: How a CEO Measures Success. In Carey D, Von Weichs M (eds.): *How to Run a Company: Lessons From Top Leaders of the CEO Academy*. New York, NY: Crown Business; 2003.
8. Ittner C, Larcker D: Coming Up Short on Nonfinancial Performance Measurement. *Harvard Business Review*. 2003; 81(11).
9. Wiig K: Knowledge Management: An Emerging Discipline Rooted in a Long History. In Depres C, Chauvel, D (eds): *Knowledge Horizons: The Present and the Promise of Knowledge Management*, Woburn, MA: Butterworth-Heinemann; 2000.

CHAPTER 9

To Centralize or Decentralize?
That Is the Question

Drexel G. DeFord, MSHI, MPA, FHIMSS, and
Dennis R. (Denny) Porter, MBA, MIS

Because this book is aimed toward the CEO, please read the following chapter with the idea that you are undertaking these improvements in your own organization. Our goal is to provide concrete concepts that can be used by the CEO to truly lead these efforts by providing scope and direction to the entire process of infrastructure management. These concepts can also be used as a basis for interviewing the information management leader that you are going to hire while going through these improvements. The CEO Crib Notes in Appendix A at the end of this chapter offer a great take-away that can be used in these real life situations.

INFORMATION TECHNOLOGY INFRASTRUCTURE: NO RESPECT

Information technology infrastructure (ITI) gets little respect from many healthcare organizations. In one of the most celebrated cases of recent times, Boston's Beth Israel Deaconess Medical Center experienced one of the worst healthcare ITI failures ever documented. For four days, the network crashed, then crashed again, and again. The network staff took what seemed to be reasonable measures to troubleshoot the problem, but the troubleshooting efforts only made the problem worse. When the root cause was finally determined, it turned out to be an antiquated network infrastructure. There was little planning or design and little or no modernization effort. Newly merged hospitals and new applications simply plugged their network into the existing Beth Israel network. Like an overloaded electrical outlet, the network finally gave up.

After 40 hours of network problems, Beth Israel went back to paper. Interns had to be taught how to write prescriptions.

What Is an Information Technology Infrastructure (ITI)?

- End-user devices (PC's, printers, etc.)
- Network servers, hardware, software, and operating systems
- Office automation products/software, including e-mail
- Personnel who plan/design/operate the utility

Automated allergy checks were lost since the system was down. Lab results that used to take minutes to come back now took hours. The risk to patient safety was increased because ITI was compromised.

"We took the plumbing for granted," said the CIO. "I was focusing on the data center. And storage growth. And after 9/11, it was backup and continuance…who thinks about the lifecycle of a switch?"[1]

ITI Is a Utility; Organizations Must Pay the Utility Bill

Depending on whom you talk to, ITI has several components including end-user devices, the network servers, hardware and operating systems, e-mail and office automation products, and the personnel who plan/design/operate ITI. Expanded definitions could include core business and clinical systems.

Just like any required utility, ITI will operate only as long as organizations pay the "utility bill." One CEO/CIO goal, then, is to make the ITI utility bill as reasonably-priced as possible. Organizations undertaking an in-depth review of their ITI management often come to realize that ITI has "grown up" over the past several years in a very "just-in-time" and disorganized way. The result is an expensive utility bill—often expensive in more ways than simple financial outlay.

Undertaking an evaluation of the current ITI management processes, then transitioning current ITI efforts (as appropriate) toward a centralized, efficient and effective organized utility operation, is one key to reducing costs and risks associated with ITI. Paying for the ITI utility as a price of business should be viewed as an unquestioned necessity. A willingness to accept marginally-controlled ITI utility bill costs should not.

FOCUSING LIMITED RESOURCES: MAKING FIRST THINGS FIRST

Healthcare exists in a resource-restricted environment. Taking a "first-things-first" approach is important. Basic management classes include studies of Maslow's hierarchy of needs. The ITI utility would be equivalent to physiological needs in Maslow's hierarchy (the lowest level need, and the one that must be reliably satisfied before those above it—safety, social, esteem, and self-actualization—can be consistently pursued). ITI would be the foundation upon which all other information projects are built. Therefore, the physiological foundation (ITI utility) must be strong and reliable. Compaq's CEO Carly Fiorina spoke to the College of Healthcare Information Management Executives, saying, "If you get the infrastructure right, everything is possible; this gives you the ability to flex to the business decisions being made."[2] Until the basic physiological information needs are met, no other organizational information needs can truly be effectively and consistently advanced.

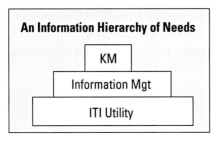

An Information Hierarchy of Needs

KM

Information Mgt

ITI Utility

Taken a step further, the Maslow analogy can be expanded beyond the ITI utility/physiological need example. Information management (IM) and knowledge management (KM) could be viewed as higher-level needs in an "information hierarchy of needs." IM, as the desire to put the right high-quality information in the right place at the right time, could comfortably sit atop ITI utility foundation. A KM layer, focused on sharing, protecting and exploiting all of a healthcare system's intellectual capital, would top IM.

Given this design, and a first-things-first approach, a healthcare organization should consider making financial investments in IT that would become part of IM and KM layers *only after* considering the impact that these procurements would have on the ITI Utility. In fact, IM/KM projects can only be considered after the ITI utility bill (consisting of refresh cycles, development and adherence to technology standards/architecture, and human resources investments) has been paid. To do otherwise is, for all intents and purposes, to plan and fund failure. IM/KM projects directed without consideration of the ITI utility are eventually doomed to failure as the ITI foundation crumbles beneath the project.

SOME WILL ARGUE: IT DOES NOT MATTER

Oddly, some will argue that IT is not really important anymore. Nicholas Carr's 2003 article in the *Harvard Business Review* entitled "I.T. Doesn't Matter" shook up many CEOs and CIOs with its provocative title and assertion that IT can no longer provide a competitive advantage.[3] For those who read past the title, and dug deeper into Carr's argument, several gems were to be discovered. The authors believe Carr to be perfectly on the mark, as far as he goes. Putting the title aside, the assertion that being so ubiquitous, ITI (emphasis on *technology*) is no longer providing a competitive advantage *in and of itself.* But while the technology no longer inherently provides a significant strategic advantage, ITI is certainly positioned to provide (in a worst case) a severe hindrance to business if it is not properly maintained and the utility bill is not paid (reference Beth Israel).[1]

Carr says that IT "wants to be shared"—as information technologies become more ubiquitous, they move from the category of "new innovations" and quickly are absorbed as part of the "utility." The competitive advantages gained by using a new piece of technology that competitors did not have or could not afford are quickly lost in today's fast-moving IT environment. Think of it this way: today's investments in IM or KM layers of the information hierarchy of needs, done to gain competitive advantage, will only provide a competitive advantage for so long if the IT itself was the advantage to be counted on. If Carr's assertions hold true, those investments may eventually (sooner rather than later) become part of an ever-growing ITI utility, no longer creating a "competitive difference" between one healthcare organization and the next. Carr's assertion only holds true if one believes technology alone is the only way to gain strategic advantage.

IF TECHNOLOGY ITSELF DOES NOT MATTER, TECHNOLOGY MANAGEMENT IS CRITICAL

ITI has become a competitive necessity, even if the technology itself is no longer providing strategic competitive advantage. Thoughts about how to invest in ITI, therefore, must change. It is time to focus on optimizing ITI and getting the most efficient, flexible, reliable utility for the least amount of money. If ITI no longer inherently offers a strategic competitive advantage, how do we *use* ITI to gain strategic competitive advantage?

Proper ITI management *may* provide spectacular cost savings, but it is not all about the money. Strong, centralized ITI management can reduce variability, improve security, reduce human resource requirements, enhance flexibility, reduce procurement costs, reduce total-cost-of-ownership, improve end-user satisfaction, and more effectively and efficiently align to business needs. Moving forward, the competitive advantage comes less and less from the purchase and installation of cutting-edge IT, and more and more through the proper management of ITI.

FROM CONFEDERATION TO FEDERATION: ADOPTING A CENTRALIZED ITI MANAGEMENT MODEL

A centralized ITI approach can work for healthcare organizations of all sizes. In general, the larger the enterprise, the more benefit financially that can be realized; however, no matter the organizational size, a centralized ITI management model will bear fruit.

> **Centralized ITI Management Approach**
>
> - Reduces variability
> - Improves security
> - Reduces human resource requirements
> - Enhances flexibility
> - Reduces procurement costs
> - Reduces total-cost-of-ownership
> - Improves end-user satisfaction
> - More effectively and efficiently align ITI to business needs

Many healthcare enterprises decentralized ITI funding to the lowest organizational level, considering this a "normal course of business." In this *decentralized* model, individual medical facilities (of all sizes) and other enterprise organizations (such as regional or corporate headquarters) solve their own ITI challenges locally. As a result, each organization wrestles with limited individual budgets. Depending on the individual organization's understanding of, and willingness to spend money on ITI, medical facilities can become either an ITI "rags" or "riches" story. From an ITI standpoint, any multi-organization healthcare enterprise dealing with ITI using this decentralized approach is, at best, a loose ITI *confederation*. A decentralized approach often results in different ITI positions for every organization in the enterprise.

Such organizational ITI variation can drastically affect the ability of the enterprise to deliver healthcare. Making "just-in-time" investments in ITI often creates unpredictable financial requirements—essentially creating unplanned financial "sine-waves" in corporate budgets.

A centralized ITI management approach, in contrast, offers the following advantages:
- Reduces variability
- Improves security
- Reduces human resource requirements
- Enhances flexibility
- Reduces procurement costs
- Reduces total-cost-of-ownership
- Improves end-user satisfaction
- More effectively and efficiently aligns ITI to business needs

So how does a healthcare enterprise make the transition from a confederated to a federated/centralized ITI approach? Often the most difficult part of the transition is simply figuring out the right way to start.

FINDING A STARTING POINT: ITI "MULTIPHASIC HEALTH SURVEY"

If one accepts the assertion that ITI can be more effectively planned, budgeted, and executed when accomplished centrally, then the first step in making the transition is to determine the enterprise's current ITI status. An ITI Multiphasic Health Survey is one way to accomplish such a benchmarking effort.

> **What does an ITI Multiphasic Health Survey ask about?**
>
> - PC fleet currently operating
> - Information about the LAN
> - IT training and certifications of personnel
> - Types of network operating systems, e-mail systems, and office automation used
> - Servers, server operating systems, and applications being used

Years ago, Dr. Morris Collin, one of the earliest medical informaticists, created a process to determine the "health status" of patients before enrolling them into a health maintenance organization.[4] His methodology classified individuals, generally, as "well," "sick," or "chronic." An ITI Multiphasic Health Survey takes a similar approach to determine ITI "health status" of each enterprise organization.

There are several acceptable approaches for accomplishing an ITI Multiphasic Health Survey, ranging from simple spreadsheets to Web surveys supported by elaborate databases. In fact, if an organization has undertaken a formal total-cost-of-ownership study for any of its technology assets, some parts of the ITI Multiphasic Health Survey are already completed. As the CEO provides the overall guidance and perspective on the process, the most important (and toughest) part of conducting this survey is determining the right questions to ask in an effort to determine ITI health status baseline.

In general, questions should focus on five ITI categories: (1) the age and processing power of the current PC inventory; (2) the status and age of network infrastructure components; (3) the types of network operating systems, e-mail systems, and office automation packages being used; (4) the number of servers being operated, the age and processing power of those servers, including a list of applications being supported; and (5) the training and certifications of the IT professionals operating the ITI.

With the data in hand, the analysis can begin. With most enterprises, initial results reveal a surprising variation in types, age, and capabilities of each of the categories listed above.

For example, organizations may discover that clinicians or medical support staff (non-IT professionals) are responsible for operating and supporting servers critical to healthcare delivery. They may find many of the servers are not secured within the confines of recognized organization or enterprise data center. It is not unusual to discover a wide variation in operating systems and brands/models of PCs being supported. The surveys can also reveal how little formal training the IT staff has and how few formal certifications they hold. The initial results of an ITI Multiphasic Health

Survey often sound the alarm—but most importantly, the analyzed results should be carefully reviewed to develop a strategy to correct the challenges identified in the survey. Which parts of ITI need the most help, and which parts need help first?

IMPLEMENTING A CENTRALIZED ITI STRATEGY: THE ROAD TO ITI WELLNESS

If the ITI Multiphasic Health Survey reveals the enterprise ITI patient is "sick," there may be several appropriate "remedies" that can be administered to bring enterprise ITI back to a healthy state. These remedies can include improving management of the network infrastructure; evaluating options of data center and server consolidation; centralized network security management; creation of a consolidated call center for troubleshooting and data analysis; and the establishment of technology refresh cycles and centralized procurement processes.

Very often, ITI Multiphasic Health Survey reveals the first step toward ITI wellness is the creation of enterprise-approved standards and architecture for hardware, software, operating systems, and personnel. If ITI is the foundation of an information hierarchy of needs, the standards and architecture rules are the "foundation-of-the-foundation."

The lack of standards unintentionally encourages ITI "hobby-shopping"—an unpredictable, expensive, and poorly managed ITI approach that often puts life-cycle management and enterprise operating capabilities at risk. Therefore, the creation of ITI standards and architecture is usually the best/first dose of medicine needed to put every organization on the path to ITI wellness.

SETTING STANDARDS, DEFINING ARCHITECTURE

Standardization is the keystone in a successful centralized ITI management approach. ITI only works right if healthcare organizations set standards and define architecture rules supporting the healthcare organization's mission. Additions to the network (including new enterprise applications) need to be engineered and planned for, not simply "plugged in." The lack of standardization significantly hampers all automation efforts including the effort to simply manage ITI. Complexity (caused by the failure to set and enforce standards) inhibits reliable and scalable ITI management.

For example, standards should be set for the types of PCs and other end-user-devices used on the network, the versions of software operating on the PCs, servers, network devices, and the model of management to be used in operating ITI. The requirement for more and more standards will become evident the deeper an organization delves into the issue. One of the goals should be to identify reduced/improved training, management, and operating costs that will result from each of the standards as they are established.

Of course, a well-understood and documented infrastructure (based on standard-setting) is critical to the long-term success of ITI. Another important point to remember throughout the effort: the standards cannot be so inflexible as to place the process above true business needs and goals; a balance must be struck.[5] In every case of standard and architecture building, additional processes must be developed to review and revise architecture standards on a regular basis. All standards must continue to evolve, in a formal and controlled manner, to support centralized ITI management and the enterprise healthcare mission requirements.

ITI standards, once invoked and coupled with ITI "refresh cycles," can be used to save money, increase end-user productivity, and create improved long-term ITI operating expense/capital investment planning and predictability.

BUILDING ITI REFRESH CYCLES AND LEVERAGING FOR REDUCED PROCUREMENT COSTS: A CENTRALIZED PC PROCUREMENT PROGRAM EXAMPLE

Many healthcare organizations do not have formal enterprise-wide "technology refresh" or replacement plans. As a result, technology refresh is often done using a "just-in-time" approach, that is, hardware or software is replaced when it fails to support the mission (this includes replacement when the item simply breaks and is no longer worth repairing). This just-in-time approach is usually on a case-by-case basis, with little thought to an enterprise-approach to lifecycle management. The approach often creates an ITI inventory which is more difficult to manage and less secure as a result. PCs are but one example of this challenge.

Desktop PCs are often pushed as far as they will go before being replaced. If funding for a new PC is not available during a budget cycle, IT directors and staff often make it through the next budget cycle by replacing PCs (via emergency purchase) as they became unrepairable. They also perform upgrades on old PCs to keep them operating. These efforts are both manpower and maintenance-fund intensive. Such costs are often hidden to organizational leadership because as a "trickle" of funds throughout the year, versus the single, large (and obvious) group inventory-replacement expenditure. When the financial "drought" continues for several years, large numbers of PCs can become outdated and more difficult for ITI staff to support, simultaneously driving down end-user productivity.

Without formal ITI refresh programs, IT directors and CIOs do not know when they will be able to replace older PCs. As a result, they often feel compelled to pay a premium price for the most cutting edge PC they can afford, when they must purchase new computers in one-at-a-time, emergency situations. They will often load up on memory and features that are "bleeding edge" technology. Why? If the machines might have to last five or six years, the reasoning goes, it needs to be as advanced as possible at the beginning of the life cycle. This practice often means organizations pay a premium price for every PC purchased. Since PCs are only purchased as they are needed, brands and models of PCs (and their operating systems) vary widely. A diverse inventory, with a multitude of brands and models, is more difficult to support than an ITI standard.

Compare this challenge to an organization with a PC technology refresh strategy aimed at replacing one-third of its inventory per year.

Using a centralized procurement approach based on a standardized PC technology refresh cycle, this scenario ensures that no PC in the inventory is more than three years old at the end of the first three (annual) replacement programs. Because PC manufacturers are willing to offer three-year warranties, this approach immediately reduces technician time and effort necessary to maintain the inventory. Support agreements became more standardized—over the course of three years, there would be, at the most, three different manufactures to call for warranty upgrade and repair.

The centralized procurement approach eliminates most of the dollars currently spent on upgrading older machines (in an effort to make them last "one more year"). This ends the costs of "throwing good money after bad." Funding is also saved on a per-PC basis because there is no longer a good reason to purchase (and pay a premium price for) a "bleeding-edge" PC as a regular practice. If the machines have to last only three years, a step back from the bleeding edge can be taken for all procurements, ensuring a relatively modern PC is always available as a client device for any application being deployed in the health system. At any point, for any project, the CIO can now readily and reliably describe the inventory, to include the oldest brand/model of PC operated, including the operating system. There are no more surprises for application developers who need to know what client-platforms operate throughout the organization.

A centralized PC procurement approach usually increases organizational average PC speed and performance, thereby reducing the time that users wait for PCs to respond to their commands/clicks. Similarly, a centralized PC procurement approach usually decreases downtime for the end-user/customer because the machines are newer and more reliable. Finally, there is the ability to centrally negotiate and execute large, bulk-procurements on a regular basis—this drives per-unit prices down even further.

Analysis at one large IDN demonstrated that this standardized/centralized procurement methodology (replacing one third of the PC inventory annually) would eliminate PC and downtime-related expenditures by approximately 20% in the first year. This IDN had been spending significant funding on upgrades and replacements without clear visibility into those expenditures. Elimination of these "cloaked" expenditures was another welcome benefit of the centralized/standardized procurement approach.

This type of ITI refresh and procurement approach can be expanded to all ITI "like items" (printers, software licenses, disposables, and so forth). By the time healthcare enterprises reach this level of ITI centralization, it is usually clear that ITI is a core requirement of the business of healthcare; that being the case, *all* ITI needs to be standardized and managed centrally as much as possible. The next several sections continue to expand on these ideals, but first, a further examination of whether an enterprise can really save money by extending the PC life cycle.

EVOLVING PC PRODUCTIVITY GAINS: CAN AN ENTERPRISE *REALLY* SAVE MONEY BY EXTENDING THE PC LIFE CYCLE?

During the 1990s, the combination of major software updates on new hardware platforms meant new PCs produced significant user-productivity gains over PCs just a year older.[6]

Today, Gartner states that the annualized total cost of ownership (TCO) for a personal computer PC kept for three years is roughly the same as for one kept for four, five or six years. However, the costs shift from direct capital and IT costs to indirect end-user costs.[7]

Enterprises should fully understand the ramifications on their total cost of ownership of keeping desktop PCs longer. Although by keeping PCs longer organizations may feel as if they are saving the enterprise money (and they actually are in some areas), they are costing the enterprise money in other areas, such as user productivity. Enterprises must understand productivity, opportunity and migration costs and come to terms with who is going to ultimately incur the costs.

A popular perception is that keeping a desktop PC after the typical three-year depreciation period is free. "The hardware is paid for, so I might as well use it as long as I can," the reasoning goes. Gartner finds that not to be the case. In fact, when the numbers were tallied, Gartner discovered that while the average annual cost of ownership for a desktop PC remains similar in the out-years, costs shift from those of direct (visible) cost categories (hardware, software and IS labor, on which the enterprise spends real currency) to categories of indirect (hidden) costs (lost end-user productivity and downtime). So, in the end, the decision comes down to one of who pays—the enterprise (in currency), or the user (in lost productivity).

Today, Gartner recommends a four-year PC lifecycle for the *mainstream* user. Enterprises must remember that keeping PCs longer than three years will result in greater hardware and operating system diversity, more software migration/licensing costs, and increased maintenance/warranty costs. Users who can find real business benefits in having a faster PC, or those who operate applications that require speedier client PCs, should opt for a shorter PC lifecycle. And something else to consider is that through 2006, 70% of all enterprises that extend desktop PC lifecycles will not achieve significant reductions in total cost of ownership.[8]

MOVING FORWARD WITH ITI CENTRALIZATION: STANDARDIZING LAN DESIGN, ENGINEERING AND INSTALLATION

Like PC purchasing, local area network (LAN) design, engineering, and installation in many healthcare systems are accomplished as a "just-in-time" program. Each facility, sometimes each department, has a different way of doing network planning and installation. This is a perfect example of "hobby-shopping," described earlier in the chapter. It is an unpredictable, expensive, and poorly managed approach that often puts life-cycle management and enterprise operating capabilities at risk. Smart "hobby-shoppers" (often not even part of the information systems department) install additional drops and expand their portions of the network haphazardly, attaching whatever devices (including medical equipment) they feel are necessary, whenever they want. Most new "hobby-shopped" network connections are simply "hung" onto existing, often weak LAN frameworks. In many enterprises, the LAN is still very much the Wild West of ITI.

Building LANs without any serious network engineering oversight, capacity planning, or design guidelines, then connecting them to an existing ITI, is the kind of approach that got Boston's Beth Israel Deaconess Medical Center in trouble.

A centralized approach to solving this challenge would involve the creation of institutional standards for local area network

> **Medical System Infrastructure Modernization (MSIM)**
>
> - Creation of a LAN "building code"
> - Goal of a "one-time" network installation taking into account future mission requirements
> - Creation of a network "sameness" from one medical facility to the next

(LAN) infrastructure, to include a formal program to pursue making these standards operational.

Such programs, sometimes referred to as medical system infrastructure modernization/management (MSIM) programs, establish guidelines to support not only design and installation processes, but also set standards for everything from a structured cable-plant cable-labeling scheme, to an acceptable drop-density in various work areas.

MSIM's standard "design-to" guidelines are much like a "building-code" for LAN installations. They ensure that all LANs are thoroughly engineered and designed networks that take all current (and anticipated future) workload and mission requirements into consideration. An MSIM program should have as one of its goals a "one-time" visit by LAN installers who completely wire facilities so that minimal (or ideally, no) "just-in-time" drops are needed when new automated information systems or network-centric medical equipment are installed. The overarching vision should be to make the network easier to understand, easier to work with, easier to maintain, and most importantly, to make the network consistently reliable for end-users.

With a skilled workforce in high demand, it is important to create network "sameness" across all medical facilities in an enterprise. Multiple benefits can result from this approach, not the least of which is a reduction of medical facility information systems staff time needed to research/trace every cable when new connections are needed. MSIM saves an incalculable number of staff hours and virtually eliminates the need for local facilities to install network cabling in a "hobby-shop" fashion.

MSIM programs can also support standardized LAN installations in new facilities as they are constructed or modified. MSIM should support all network-type expansion projects—for example, telephony upgrades. Over time, MSIM projects can evolve in the way engineering, design, and installation is accomplished (in-house resources versus outsourced). No matter what the approach, it is very important to closely control installation quality in this valuable program.

Like all other centralized/standardized ITI projects, MSIM programs must develop plans for technology refresh cycles, including LAN electronics and cabling replacement. Also like other centralized/standardized ITI programs, MSIM offers the capability of leveraging bulk purchase power with vendors. By managing LANs from an enterprise-wide approach, healthcare organizations have the ability to secure best pricing for electronics, cabling, and other installation materials.

In our experience, MSIM programs can demonstrate 50% savings on network electronics purchases (when compared to list prices), 20% savings on engineering costs (co-source versus outsourced methodology), and 10 to 30% savings on installation material (cables, racks, and the like). It is virtually impossible to calculate the human resource savings for information system organizations at the medical facility level. Likewise, it is impossible to determine how much network downtime, and resultant business impact, is cost-avoided by taking an MSIM approach to the LAN portion of ITI. One thing is clear: MSIM programs, where they exist, endure as cost-saving models for LAN infrastructure engineering, design, and deployment.

CENTRALIZING LAN MAINTENANCE; REDUCING COSTS

At the same time facilities are growing more dependent upon their ITI, the maintenance of the LAN hardware and "internetwork operating systems" (the software that runs on the LAN hardware and allows it to function optimally) is often handled in a very inconsistent way. Many medical facilities or departments purchase LAN maintenance contracts for their "piece" of the network. Worse yet, others simply have no LAN maintenance contracts of any type. Continuing down the path of centralization, the most obvious solution is to centrally purchase maintenance for all LAN components, enterprise-wide, in a single contract. Options for these programs are many, but they primarily fall into two categories: vendor maintenance contracts, or third-party integrator maintenance contracts.

To begin, organizations should develop an estimate of what they should expect to pay for LAN maintenance. For example, given one scenario for estimated coverage and response time desired, Orans[9] predicts Maintenance Charges to Installed Base (MCIB) should be about 10% of the total list price of the equipment being covered under the contract.

Careful evaluation of in-house resources (for example, engineers also assigned to work MSIM programs) and in-depth evaluation of acceptable risk can reveal less expensive alternatives to standard vendor maintenance contracts. Facilities with strong MSIM programs can often accept higher risk, because their LAN installation and engineering quality and refresh/modernization methodology provides greater confidence in long-term network reliability. Instead of manufacturer maintenance contracts, enterprises with strong MSIM programs will choose maintenance and sparing (M&S) contracts through third-party vendor/integrators. This integrator can in turn help leverage relationships with various LAN equipment manufacturers.

> **How Do I Calculate Maintenance Charge to Installed Base?**
>
> Simply divide the vendor's annual maintenance charges by the total cost of the installed base at list price.[9]

As with everything in the centralized ITI approach, serious consideration should be given to all options, with the goal being a lower utility bill (i.e., lowered financial outlay, decreased unscheduled downtime, and increased network availability and reliability to all end-users).

SERVER AND DATA CENTER CONSOLIDATION: THE LONG RUN TOWARD AN APPLICATION PORTAL

Server centralization and consolidation is yet another step toward more effective and efficient management of ITI resources in the centralized/federated model.

Servers are often drastically underutilized. One CIO relates the story of his first visit to the data center just after taking a new position. He asked about the server capacity being utilized on a particular piece of hardware. It turned out the server was running at about 5% of capacity. When he asked the same question about the other 30 servers running in the data center, the answer was similar for each. As someone once said, the underutilization of servers in today's decentralized data centers is a monument to vendors' superb marketing capability. The desire to get the most bang for the buck in the data center environment often ignites data-center and server-consolidation projects.

Data center/server consolidation projects may also reveal another little secret: Some percentage of the total server inventory may not be operating within the confines and security of a designated organization data-center at all! Finding these servers, then moving them to a data-center, is a very important part of server-consolidation efforts. Just as important is making sure these mission-critical servers have the proper "care and feeding" including security, backups, and the like. This type of consolidation effort—"backward consolidation"[10]—is essentially aimed at rounding up "orphaned" servers, mitigating the propagation of servers, and building best practices to support on-going server-consolidation.

Once servers have been consolidated into data-centers, enterprises should review ways to reduce both the number and types of servers. CIOs should work closely with automated information system developers and vendors, pushing them toward alliances that will allow for shared-hosting capabilities (putting multiple applications on a single server). Such efforts can not only reduce the number of servers in use, but also drive higher utilization of the equipment in service.

Next, enterprises should consider ways to reduce the number of data-centers housing this equipment. Core application (file and print sharing servers and the like) and other network servers can be consolidated across data centers. Data center consolidation usually happens in phases. First, the project consolidates data-centers within a given facility. Once this step is complete, future efforts focus on elimination of facility-level data-centers in favor of regional, national, or worldwide data-centers.

As part of data center consolidation, some enterprises have undertaken considerable efforts to make all applications Web-based, more capable, and more tolerant of network delays. The effort to design new applications to run in a consolidated environment, and the ability to use consolidation capability as a decision factor when purchasing new applications is known as "forward consolidation." The goal is to drive a reduction in the number of servers and data centers necessary to support an enterprise.[10] Using this model, the ultimate goal of an organization might be to have all applications available via a single user-portal, with a single user sign-on, running on a small group of servers, all in a single data center. Realizing this sort of vision may take years, but many complex healthcare organizations believe such efforts will continue to pay off.

While all data center and server consolidation efforts are aimed at reducing total cost of ownership (some enterprises have reported millions of dollars in savings), each type of consolidation offers different savings potential, with seventy percent of the savings usually coming from reduced staffing requirements. Other savings should also be considered, including the reduction in hardware, software licenses, facilities (data-center elimination), power-consumption, and the like.[11] A primary benefit, standardization, should not be overlooked in the drive to show cost-savings in server-consolidation projects.

CENTRALIZING NETWORK SECURITY

Centralization holds an additional extremely positive advantage: security. Reducing the number of servers through consolidation also reduces the number of network devices that must be monitored and "patched" by security personnel as new security software bugs are discovered and exploited by hackers.

One model holds that centralized management of a decentralized security infrastructure (firewalls, servers, clients, and intrusion detection systems) offers greater consistency of technical security policy. This consistency is gained, in part, by both reducing the number of technical security experts on staff, while maintaining each individual security "site" from a centralized location. This centralized network operations security center (CNOSC) uses remote control processes to continuously monitor network traffic and apply a standard security profile to every item in the network defense inventory.

Another model/approach to centralized network security is a centralized management of a centralized security infrastructure. Organizations using this model have actually been able to reduce the number of firewalls, servers, and other security suite devices (in effect, this is another form of server consolidation). Most often, this is accomplished through the creation of a virtual private network with reduced external "entry points" into the enterprise network. If everything inside the network is trusted, then only the entry points need to be zealously protected. In this scenario, an improved security profile (where the primary threat is considered external to the organization) can be achieved.

There should logically be a reduction in cost in both models, but many factors affect how much can be saved through consolidation (see "Some of the 'Cons' of Centralization" below). Fewer security sites and a reduced amount of equipment needing constant security updates may equate to fewer dollars spent on security. Depending on the aggressiveness of centralization and consolidation efforts, fewer personnel should be necessary to maintain technical security operations.

There are several possible uses for the resultant savings but one in particular stands out: leading organizations use the savings to hire higher-quality, credentialed technical security operators for their centralized operations. Having security experts not only maintain profiles but build protocols to deal with intrusions, monitor and mitigate vendor and product security holes as they are reported and take an active posture in defending the network, inside and out, reduces organizational costs while improving an organization's security profile.

REDUCING PERSONNEL COSTS THROUGH CENTRALIZED CALL-CENTERS AND OTHER OPERATIONS

As alluded to in the previous section, centralization can position enterprises to save money in one very expensive area of the business: personnel. By centralizing, organizations may be able to reduce the number of personnel involved in ITI operation, while simultaneously improving the standardization and operation of the ITI utility.

At the management level, larger organizations taking a centralized approach are often able to eliminate CIO positions at the medical facility level. Many of the duties and responsibilities previously managed by a facility CIO have migrated to regional CIOs, or have been assumed by a centralized corporate staff managing enterprise procurement processes, data analysis, servers, networks, and security challenges.

Some of the most heavily centralized enterprises have taken the logical step of centralizing ITI helpdesk into a central call-center. All customer calls are directed to a staff of technicians who handle most of the troubleshooting and repairs remotely, using remote management tools to "reach through the network" and repair affected device, load software, or update necessary drivers. These approaches have greatly reduced the need for "hands-on" technician support at the site. Calls are triaged through a variety of levels, depending upon the problem, to technical or application experts who work hard to resolve those problems remotely (Figure 9-1).

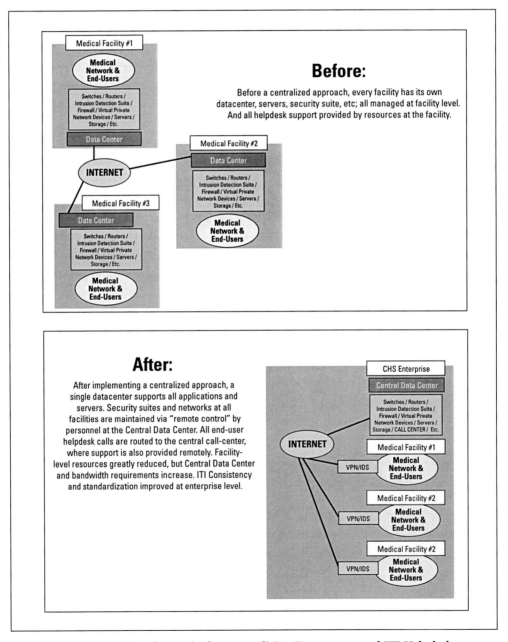

Figure 9-1. Before and After Centralizing Datacenters and ITI Helpdesks

Remote troubleshooting has reduced the number of technicians necessary at the facility level. Remaining technicians are used as the last line of defense for helpdesk calls that cannot be resolved remotely. The technicians work closely with the central helpdesk to troubleshoot and document ways to improve "remote-control" customer service. They also support replacement and testing of end-user devices (PCs and printers, for example) and network components. The need for large, decentralized IT staffs with broad/extensive knowledge can be reduced using a centralized ITI approach because the centralized staff has a larger area of responsibility and can more consistently resolve nearly all common customer issues.

In this centralized scenario, regional and corporate staffs may grow, but overall total staff numbers will likely be reduced. One large IDN has been able to reduce total information systems department FTEs to 150, while supporting nearly 1,700 facilities worldwide.

A centralized approach can also improve data analysis and reporting of both clinical and business data. Server consolidation has naturally led to data consolidation, with fewer datasets to be mined. Because of this, organizations can employ fewer, more experienced analysts. With centralization, a system-wide view of business/clinical trends can be identified more easily; this can create an enterprise-wide problem-solving approach, saving money, and improving healthcare delivery.

SOME OF THE CONS OF CENTRALIZATION

Of course, centralization of ITI is not without its drawbacks. Here are a few of the pitfalls that must be carefully considered when moving to a centralized ITI approach.

Centers of Gravity

Centralization of data centers and security management, standardization of applications enterprise-wide, and centralization of personnel expertise, especially at a single physical location, creates a center of gravity. A disruption of any sort, large or small at this centralized operating location can cause chaos. Weather, natural disaster, or homeland defense challenges create a huge requirement for redundant capabilities, contingency operations (COOP) plans, and data and server back-up sites. These COOP and back-up plans become incredibly important when operating in a very centralized model. In a large IDN, failure of a centralized site affects the whole enterprise. The plans must be tested regularly and rigorously to ensure business and healthcare continuity.

Wide Area Network Reliability

Centralization of applications, data centers, and the like, means not only is the local area network part of ITI, the wide area network now becomes a critical part of ITI. Wide-area connectivity (connectivity between operating locations not on in the same building or on the same campus) is often much more difficult to control. This kind of connectivity requires significant engineering and design effort to be put against the requirement, so proper redundancy, alternate data flow, and network capability can be ensured.

Centralization Landmines
• Centers of gravity • Wide area network reliability • One-size-fits-all • "Consistency" cuts both ways • Third-party integrator maintenance is not perfect • Data-center and server-consolidation savings can be elusive • Not all the bad-guys are outside your network

One Size Fits All

The belief that "one-size-fits-all" can be a seriously negative side effect to centralized ITI management. Once centralized, corporate managers will decide what is best for an enterprise. While this consistency of thought has many positive aspects, it can also generate dreadful results. Not every medical facility in an enterprise is exactly the same size, nor does it have exactly the same need. There may have to be multiple ITI "solution sets" for various categories of facilities (based on size, mission, or other criteria). Failure to avoid a one-size-fits-all mentality will result in over- or under-spending to support facilities. Even worse, it can result in over- or under-capability for a facility trying to use ITI to deliver critically important healthcare.

The more centralized procurement efforts become, the more important it is to have input and buy-in from the end-users (or their representatives) at each facility. Not everything lends itself to centralized procurement methodology. If a healthcare organization is only planning on purchasing a small number of low-cost "widgets" this year, maybe it is best to leave that procurement decentralized. There may be little or no volume discount on such a purchase.

Consistency Cuts Both Ways

Consistency through centralization can be a huge security benefit, but it may also create a very dangerous flaw. Centralized management of multiple security sites may lead to a very consistent profile, but if the profile is flawed (i.e., there is a security hole), that flaw will be present at every location.

Third-Party Integrator Maintenance Requires Research

On the issue of using third-party integrators to support ITI maintenance and sparing efforts, while funding can be reduced in many cases, there can be some drawbacks. CIOs must realize that using a third-party vendor is not the same as having direct access to the manufacturer's support team. The integrator approach is, in fact, one step removed from direct manufacturer support. Careful evaluation of the integrator's relationship with ITI equipment manufacturers is a very important part of the analysis when deciding how best to deal with local area network maintenance and sparing.

Data-Center and Server-Consolidation Savings Can Be Elusive

Shared hosting continues to prove extremely difficult. Think of it this way. Each application is a family living together in a single-family home (the server). As an enterprise consolidates servers, shared hosting is much like asking the families to cohabitate in a single large building (often without walls). Sometimes the families find it difficult to live in such close proximity to each other. Applications also have the same problems learning to live inside a single server. A survey of data center managers confirmed that shared-hosting is one of the most-desired future server capabilities.[12]

As a matter of fact, server consolidation in general continues to be one of the toughest issues facing enterprises today. In some cases, bandwidth to consolidate simply is not available in some areas. In other projects, savings expected from server consolidation had to be spent on additional corporate centralized data center capabilities or other central management tools. Software vendor pricing scenarios can also drive software license costs up in "per-processor" pricing scenarios. While most often this scenario provides an incentive to consolidate when multiple copies of the same software stack can be consolidated onto larger systems with fewer total processors, the scenario can turn ugly when trying different software stacks onto larger servers. If the software vendor does not take consolidation efforts into consideration when developing pricing schemes, some server consolidation efforts could be subject to this hidden cost.[10]

Many other factors can affect expected server consolidation savings, making a project that is worthwhile for a multitude of reasons appear to be a business failure. Enterprises savings have been extremely variable for several reasons: the number and utilizations of the servers being targeted, the type of platform (mainframe, Unix, Windows, Linux), the type of software contracts, the age and disposition of equipment, and the disposition of staff are just a few of the variables that can greatly affect the outcome of server consolidation projects. Consistent, secure, reliable server operation may be hard to "price," but these soft costs can make a server consolidation project more than worthwhile.[13]

Not All the "Bad Guys" Are Outside the Network

From the standpoint of security, remember that much of the threat continues to be from inside the network.[14] Zealously protecting the entry-points of a network from outside intruders may give a false sense of security. Good overall security policy is necessary to protect the network from the inside out.

WHERE TO FROM HERE?

As the CEO and leader of the organization, you set the tone and direction for all change. It is to be hoped that you have gathered some points that will assist you in the vital role of senior leadership guiding infrastructure management. The truth is that ITI in most healthcare organizations has grown up willy-nilly over the past several years. A just-in-time cornucopia of products, network installations, and security gear has satisfied immediate needs, often with no long-term view of how to prepare for the future.

ITI is a huge investment. There is no better time than the present to begin the process of wringing out the best value of every dollar being spent—paying the ITI utility bill. So, go ahead, set ITI refresh cycles. Build architectural standards and stand behind them. Train and retrain the staff that designs/installs/maintains the ITI utility. Experienced professionals with an understanding of both technology and healthcare are the most vital part of ITI. Drive hard toward centralization and consolidation, but remember, it can't always be about "hard" savings.

In the end, your centralization efforts will pay off in all sorts of ways. Most importantly, ITI will have the respect and attention it deserves, and you will be rewarded with an increase in ITI flexibility and security, a decrease in ITI complexity, and improved customer service across the board.

APPENDIX A:
CEO CRIB NOTES LEADING INFRASTRUCTURE MANAGEMENT

- What is information technology infrastructure (ITI)?
  - End-user devices
  - Network hardware/software/operating systems
  - Office automation products/e-mail
  - Personnel who plan/design/operate ITI
  - (Definition can be expanded as desired)

- ITI is a utility; organizations must pay the utility bill

- But resources are limited: how to focus on "first things first?"
  - "Information hierarchy of needs" model: ITI is the foundation of much of today's healthcare business
  - Organizations must focus on optimizing ITI and getting the most efficient, flexible, reliable utility for the least amount of money

- Some will argue: information technology doesn't matter…

- …If the technology itself doesn't matter, then the way technology is managed is critical
  - Proper ITI management *may* provide spectacular cost savings, but it's not all about the money.
  - Strong, centralized ITI management can:
    - Reduce variability
    - Improve security
    - Reduce human resource requirements
    - Enhance flexibility
    - Reduce procurement costs
    - Reduce total-cost-of-ownership
    - Improve end-user satisfaction
    - More effectively and efficiently align ITI to business needs
  - Today, competitive advantage comes less and less from the purchase and installation of cutting-edge IT, and more and more from the proper management of ITI

- Adopting a centralized ITI management model avoids:
  - ITI variation at the organizational level
  - Unplanned, just-in-time ITI financial investments

- Getting started: accomplish an ITI "multiphasic health survey" for all facilities
  - Discover information about end-user devices
  - Discover information about local area network hardware/software
  - Determine training & certifications of IT professionals
  - Determine types of systems/software used in the enterprise
  - Determine number/types of servers, operating systems, and applications used in the enterprise

- Implementing a centralized ITI strategy; getting on the road to ITI "wellness"
  - Establish standards and define architecture

- Build ITI refresh cycles
- Leverage standards and refresh cycles to reduce procurement costs of PCs, printers, and like items
- Standardize the design/installation/management/maintenance of local area network infrastructure
- Take steps toward data center and server consolidation
- Centralize network security management through a centralized network operations security center (CNOSC)
- Build a single corporate call center for enterprise operations supporting remote system troubleshooting/repair and centralized business and clinical data analysis

• Centralization is not without its pitfalls: remember to watch out for the following dangers:
  - "Center of gravity"
  - Wide-area network reliability
  - "One-size-fits-all"
  - Consistency cuts both ways
  - Third-party integrator maintenance is not perfect
  - Data-center and server-consolidation savings can be elusive
  - Not all the bad guys are outside your network

Drexel G. DeFord, MSH, MPA, FHIMSS, is the Chief Technology Officer for the U.S. Air Force Medical Service, a $6.2 billion globally distributed healthcare system with over 39,000 employees and 74 hospitals and clinics. During his 19-year military career, he has served as a Regional Chief Information Officer, a Medical Center Chief Information Officer, and has completed two tours in Southwest Asia, including Operations Desert Shield and Desert Storm. He is a Fellow in HIMSS, where he serves as the Chair of the Microsoft Healthcare Users' Group Board of Directors, and as an advisory member to the HIMSS Board of Directors. He holds masters degrees in both public administration and health informatics.

Dennis R. (Denny) Porter, MBA, MIS, is a senior executive in Integic's Health-Care Practice Area. Throughout a healthcare career spanning more than 25 years he has served in a variety of business executive leadership roles, including Chief Information Officer. He is one of nine national leaders serving on the HIMSS Electronic Health Record Steering Committee. Mr. Porter earned a masters degree in business administration management information systems from Oklahoma City University.

References

1. Berinato S: All Systems Down. *CIO Magazine*. February 25, 2003.
2. Fiorina C: Keynote Address to the College of Healthcare Information Management Executives Conference, San Diego, California; February 9, 2003.
3. Carr NG: IT Doesn't Matter. *Harvard Business Review*. May, 2003.
4. Collin MF: *A History of Medical Informatics in the United States*. Indianapolis, IN: American Medical Informatics Association; 1995.
5. Colville R, Scott D: Client Issues for IT Operations Architecture. Gartner Key Issues, K-21-1432. September 30, 2003.

6. Margevicius MA: Desktop PC Life: Four Years for the Mainstream. Gartner Note Number T-13-8045; August 21, 2001.

7. Tonneson B, Escherich M: *Hardware Platforms Weekly.* No. 38; September 29, 2003.

8. Silver M, Federica T: Desktop TCO for Years 4, 5, and 6: Someone Has to Pay. Gartner Note Number: SPA-20-5018; September 9, 2003.

9. Orans L: Three Steps to Lower Network Maintenance Charges. Gartner Tactical Guidelines; TG-10-9466; 2000.

10. Chuba M, Phelps JR: Will Consolidation Still Be a Hot Topic in 2006? Gartner Note Number COM-19-7922; May 19, 2003.

11. Phelps JR: Consolidating Servers Cuts TCO Significantly – Sometimes. Gartner Note Number DF-15-6463; March 15, 2002.

12. Bittman TJ: Users Say Consolidation Is Top Windows Server Issue. Gartner Note Number COM-19-8828; May 8, 2002.

13. Phelps, John R: (2003, May 13), Many Factors Affect Server Consolidation Savings. Gartner Note Number COM-19-5851; May 13, 2003.

14. Computer Security Institute; Federal Bureau of Investigations (CSI/FBI); Computer Crime and Security Survey; 2003.

Epilogue

John P. Glaser, PhD, FCHIME, FHIMSS

CHAPTER 1: IT GOVERNANCE

Sam was pleased with the work they had done on IT governance. A Steering Committee had been formed and its role had been defined. The Ingalls leadership was on board and his CIO had begun to develop the agenda for the meetings ahead.

Sam did not doubt that the Committee would have difficult discussions and that his skill would be required to lead the group to make some complex and critical decisions on the IT direction, IT budget and vendor selection. However, the governance mechanisms that they had established would serve them well.

CHAPTER 2: WIREHEADS AND TECHNOPHOBES

Sam realized that he often experienced communication issues in his interactions with the medical and administrative staff. A junior administrator might not have had enough experience to know how to phrase suggestions at department head meetings. The CFO would wander into arcane details of Medicare reimbursement. Some members of his team would hold back in expressing their true reservations about a proposal.

Improving communication in those cases, and with his CIO, would require coaching. It would require that Sam stop the person and ask them to "explain it in English." It would involve ensuring that individuals spend time in meetings or other settings in which they would be immersed (and hopefully absorb) the language used by the leadership team. And it would involve using techniques such as vision statements and communication plans.

While improving the communication skills of the CIO would require work on his part and the CIO's, Sam knew that this would be worth the effort.

CHAPTER 3: ART OF BUSINESS AND IT STRATEGIC ALIGNMENT

Sam found the IT alignment discussion to be one of the most important in his career. He now understood that alignment needed a senior leadership discussion that clarified the goals and strategies of the organization and that the IT strategy was intertwined in those discussions. He now realized that the team had to ask, during strategy discussions, how will our IT investments help us to achieve our goals?

Sam realized that the goals for the IT agenda were not something that they should delegate solely to the CIO. Rather, the discussion of IT goals was a discussion that involved all of the leadership.

Sam now knew that the entire leadership team shared the accountability for the results of the IT investments. Accountability was not something that the team could place entirely on the shoulders of the IT organization.

Finally, Sam realized that he needed to spend time with his CIO. Sam had to help his CIO understand Sam's perspectives on leadership, IT, the challenges faced by the organization, and the power of treating users as customers. Alignment was more than linking IT to the organization's strategies; it also involved the CEO and CIO understanding each other's views of the industry and the organization.

CHAPTER 4: GETTING VALUE FROM YOUR IT INVESTMENTS

Sam was not particularly happy with the realization that IT value was multi-faceted and often soft. However, he realized that Ingalls would be able to do a good job prioritizing IT projects using formal criteria supplemented by, as they often had to do with other resource decisions, judgment and instinct.

More importantly, Sam planned to use an upcoming leadership retreat to develop a series of management processes and steps designed to ensure that they realized IT value: auditing the value of completed IT initiatives, ensuring accountability for results, assessing their IT investments as a portfolio and strengthening the IT proposal process. In particular, Sam wanted to engage his team in a discussion of steps to reduce the impact of IT value dilution factors.

CHAPTER 5: ASSESSING YOUR IT ORGANIZATION'S PERFORMANCE

Sam knew that his IT organization was not perfect. And despite the boasting of some of his colleagues on the east coast, he knew that their organizations were not perfect either. But he believed that he was now in a much better position to understand the critical areas of IT performance and determine whether the performance was acceptable or not.

The discussion he had had with his management team about IT performance measures had been both important and useful. The group had come to consensus on the critical performance areas and the right way to measure or assess those areas.

Sam was looking forward to the development of the resulting IT performance dashboard. He knew that not all of the areas were amenable to numeric scores. Nonetheless, Ingalls now had a framework of critical questions for assessing IT. Sam planned to review that dashboard and the more qualitative responses to the questions in his meetings with the CIO and at the quarterly meeting of the larger management team.

Sam also realized that IT performance was a responsibility shared between IT and the rest of the leadership team.

CHAPTER 6: OUTSOURCING AND THE MERITS OF MARRIAGE

Sam had realized that outsourcing was not some form of management silver bullet—it would not cure all IT aliments. Outsourcing was a complex and difficult management decision, a decision that had to be approached in phases and with respect for the significance of the undertaking.

Sam also appreciated that outsourcing was not an all-or-nothing proposition. The organization could outsource the entire IT department but it could also outsource specific functions such as management of the network and the data center.

Sam did not doubt the claims that he had read about outsourcing. But now he also did not believe that those gains were inherent with outsourcing or that they were easily achieved. He decided to keep outsourcing as an option and to spend some time, in the months ahead, gaining a deeper understanding of the topic.

CHAPTER 7: THE CEO-CIO RELATIONSHIP

Sam decided that he would change the focus of the next several meetings that he was scheduled to have with the CIO. Rather than talk about budgets and project status, he and the CIO would talk about their relationship and how to make it work better. Sam wanted to discuss what each of them believed was the basis of a good working relationship and if their relationship needed some work in areas such as communication or respect, then the two of them would commit to doing that work.

Sam believed that they should both talk about what each expected from the other and Sam would candidly talk about the attributes and skills that he would like to see in the CIO. People have to work on their relationships and have the honest discussions needed to identify problems and hold each other accountable for taking whatever steps they both decided need to occur.

Sam thought that he would also take the CIO to a basketball game and take some time to get to know each other better.

CHAPTER 8: BUILDING A KNOWLEDGE-ENABLED ORGANIZATION

Sam was startled to realize that, although all of the management and medical staff leadership regarded data and information as an important organizational asset, Ingalls did not manage that asset comprehensively and consistently.

While he still had more to learn about information management, he was convinced that the organization needed to begin to pursue best practices in this area; strategic data mapping, data warehousing, digital performance dashboards, central support and management of these activities, data mining, knowledge management, and enterprise portals.

Information management might not be as sexy as state-of-the-art IT but Sam thought it might be more important.

CHAPTER 9: TO CENTRALIZE OR DECENTRALIZE?

Sam still believed that he was never going to be a techno-phile. But he felt a lot more comfortable with the discussion surrounding IT infrastructure.

He understood that Ingalls needed central control and management of the infrastructure just as Ingalls needed central management of finance. He appreciated the need for infrastructure standards just as the organization needed standards in human resource recruiting, merit programs and benefits. He knew that the infrastructure would need to be technically refreshed just as the physical plant needed periodic refreshing.

Sam appreciated that any centralization carried with it concerns and challenges. A management team could over centralize anything and create problems as it was trying to solve problems.

Sam also had developed a better understanding of the importance and role of elements of the infrastructure such as networks, security and servers. He was not ready to become a programmer but he was ready to engage the CIO and the management team in the infrastructure discussion.

POSTSCRIPT

Tired from the day, Sam decided to head home, ignoring the pile of papers and e-mail that awaited his attention. Tomorrow he was going to have to begin to spend more time on the IT issues of Ingalls.

Some changes would need to be made if they were to improve the organization's use of IT. However, Sam felt that he had a much better understanding of the nature of the IT challenge and the steps that the organization would have to take. A lot of progress had been made—not a bad day's work.

Index

reasons for, 88
selection criteria, 90–92

P

PC life cycles, 142–143
Performance assessment, 75–86, 158. *See also* Information systems
    alternative management, 84–85
    future concerns, 85
    productivity and cost management, 84
    project management, 82–83
    staff development, 83
    strategic planning, 81–82
    system availability, 77
    system protection, 80–81
    system reliability, 78
    system security, 81
    usability, 78–80
    vendor/contract management, 85
Project management, 82–83

R

Reflective knowledge management, 127
Return on investment (ROI), 56–57, 59

S

Security and firewalls, 80, 81, 146–147
Shared accountability, 43–45
    examples of, 44–45
Strategic alignment, 39–51, 157–158
    CEO perspective, 45–49
    characteristics of IT executives, 47–49
    definition of, 41
    expectations, 49
    and planning, 81–82
    process for, 49
    shared accountability, 43–45
    synergy of purpose, 41–43
Staff development, 83
Strategic data mapping, 116–118
    creation of, 117
    enterprise performance measurement, 117–118

T

Technophobia reduction, 21–23
    and acquisition processes, 22
    communication plan, 22
    media use, 21
    strategic planning sessions, 22
    and technology assessment committees, 23
    vision setting, 21–22
Training of staff, 83
Transactional knowledge management, 126–127

V

Value of information technology, 53–72
    delivery of, 66–72
    effectiveness, 62–65
    investment failures, 58–62
    IT proposals, 55
    nature of, 54–58
    problems of, 53–54
    single investments, 55–56
Vendor management, 85

W

Web portals, 127–128
Wireless access, 79